American Nursing

American Nursing:
From Hospitals to Health Systems

Joan E. Lynaugh, Ph.D., FAAN

and

Barbara L. Brush, Ph.D., RN

A Copublication with the Milbank Memorial Fund

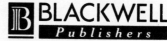

First published 1996
Reprinted 1998

Blackwell Publishers Inc
350 Main Street
Malden, Massachusetts 02148, USA

Blackwell Publishers Ltd
108 Cowley Road
Oxford OX4 1JF, UK

Library of Congress Cataloging in Publication Data has been applied for

British Library Cataloguing in Publication Data
A CIP catalogue record for this book is available from the British Library

ISBN 1–57718–046–1 (pbk)

Copublished by Milbank Memorial Fund
Printed in Great Britain by Athenæum Press Ltd, Gateshead, Tyne & Wear

This book is printed on acid-free paper

Contents

Abbreviations

AACN	American Association of Critical-Care Nurses
AANA	American Association of Nurse Anesthetists
ADN	Associate Degree Nurse
AMA	American Medical Association
ANA	American Nurses Association
BSN	Bachelor of Science in Nursing
DHEW	Department of Health Education and Welfare
DHHS	Department of Health and Human Services
DRG	Diagnostically Related Groups
EVP	Exchange Visitor Program
HEW	Health, Education and Welfare
ICU	Intensive Care Unit
IOM	Institute of Medicine
JAHA	*Journal of the American Hospital Association*
JAMA	*Journal of the American Medical Association*
LPNs	Licensed Practical Nurses
NACG	National Association of Colored Graduates
NJPC	National Joint Practice Commission
NLN	National League for Nursing
NLNE	National League for Nursing Education
NNC	National Nursing Council
NOPHN	National Organization of Public Health Nursing

ONS   Oncology Nursing Society
PHS   Public Health Service
PNA   Pennsylvania Nurses Association
PPC   Progressive Patient Care
RN   Registered Nurse
USDHEW   United States Department of Health Education and Welfare
USGPO   United States Government Printing Office
USPHS   United States Public Health Service
WHO   World Health Organization
WICHE   Western Interstate Commission for Higher Education

Preface

American nurses in the 1990s are different in character, appearance, and circumstance from their predecessors who lived and worked in the 1940s. This transformation is manifested in their education, clinical responsibility and, of course, in the huge increase in their numbers relative to the population. During recent decades the scope of nurses' practice has expanded to include many new responsibilities, including work formerly in the province of physicians, as well as entirely new functions. More nurses who hold professional licenses now have more general and specialized education than did their counterparts of the 1940s and 1950s. Today, however, the term "nurse" encompasses a wider and more complex spectrum of individual academic attainment and practice than was true in 1950. In the 1980s nurses began to be much better paid relative to previous decades and to other workers. Taken together, all these factors add up to new and different life-style and career prospects associated with nursing.[1]

But, in some senses, this forty-year period in nursing history is as much a story of the metamorphosis in hospitals as one of change in nursing. A colleague argues, "there has been no policy [for nursing] other than that which supports the survival and growth of hospitals."[2] She makes a vital point, for the centrality of the hospital to our health-care system reached its fullest expression and remained unchallenged through these years of nursing expansion. However, hospitals are changing too. The last forty years frames an intriguing period which includes both the apex of centralization of care in hospitals and the beginning of a transition toward decentralizing care out of hospitals. As we near the end of the twentieth century more of the sick, injured, and dependent will be nursed in their homes or in other less complex and costly institutions. The relocation of nurses' work is a crucial part of this decentralization. As health-care systems organize to emphasize care in the community, the home, and other alternative settings, the centrality of the hospital to the system and to nursing will probably be diminished.

The Historical Context

Since the nineteenth century nurses and hospitals have shared a relationship seemingly indispensable to both occupation and institution. Nurses' work keeps hospitals functioning; hospitals provide nurses with employment and a base for their practice. This relationship, often plagued with difficulty, is now caught up in the sweeping changes in the health-care environment. This book focuses on the most recent fifty years of the hospital–nursing history looking at some of the main events and issues of a very complex relationship.

To date no single secondary source reports on this highly eventful, sometimes tumultuous era in nursing. A rapidly growing professional literature and an almost constant barrage of commissioned studies of nursing during the period of study, however, have provided more than ample material for reconsideration and analysis of the linkages between nursing and hospitals.

Scholarship on earlier nursing history can be found in the work of Susan Reverby, Barbara Melosh, Nancy Tomes, and Celia Davis, among others.[3] They make clear that, before and immediately after World War II, most nurse caregivers in hospitals were pupil nurses supervised by a few fully trained graduate nurses. Indeed, the training schools and their pupils were crucial to hospital development as a source of labor. After World War II hospitals finally began to employ fully trained nurses and their assistants as caregivers for most patients. The spectrum of problems and issues stemming from this change as well as the broader changes in the American health-care system prompted this study.

Historians have subjected American hospitals to considerable scrutiny in recent years. Morris Vogel, Charles Rosenberg, Rosemary Stevens and David Rosner, among others, investigated and analyzed the important symbolic, scientific, economic, and service role played by hospitals in America's towns and cities.[4] The interest of scholars and the public in hospitals and their history in our communities is due, in no small measure, to the pervasive sense that today's hospitals are troubled institutions.

Four issues dominated more than two generations of debate about nursing: the nature, scope and quality of nursing practice; the means of educating nurses; authority relationships among nurses, physicians and hospital administrators; and recurring complaints of a shortage of hospital nurses. Most studies of "nursing" actually focused on hospital needs for nurses rather than on nursing as a discipline or general public service. This particular history of nursing holds hospitals central and influential as a context for analysis.

The text is arranged chronologically. It begins with the hospital-building period between the end of World War II and the mid-sixties. The pattern of paid hospital nursing staff was developed during this era. Next we examine nursing's radical expansion between 1965 and 1983 when payment for hospital care was transformed, first by Medicare and Medicaid and then by prospective reimbursement organized around the concept of diagnostically related groups (DRGs). We conclude with the round of national studies of nursing commissioned in the 1980s and early 1990s and the commentary they inspired. Finally, we offer some observations and recommendations based on our interpretation of events in the history of hospital nursing and American health care since World War II.

We are indebted to our colleagues Ellen D. Baer, Karen Buhler-Wilkerson, and Julie Fairman at the Center for the Study of the History of Nursing, University of Pennsylvania School of Nursing, for their many suggestions and helpful criticisms. Distinguished nurses and historians substantially improved our thinking by their informed and helpful readings. Finally, we are most appreciative of the support of the Milbank Memorial Fund for this undertaking.

Bureaucratizing Care, 1945–1960

Hospitals and Nursing after World War II

We immediately think of women in white – graduate nurses – when we picture the rooms and corridors of hospitals, but the phenomenon of fully prepared nurses as hospital employees is relatively recent. Three-quarters of all graduate nurses in the 1920s and early 1930s were concentrated in the private duty market, working either in patients' homes or as "specials" for patients requiring hospitalization. These graduate nurses were paid by the patients they cared for, usually on a daily or weekly basis. It was student nurses who were the mainstay workforce for hospitals; graduate nurses' work was not intrinsically linked to the hospital ward until the 1940s.[5]

The transition of nurses from home to hospital, however, was not all-inclusive. Though 53 percent of white nurses were employed in hospitals in 1948, black nurses, who comprised 2 percent of the total registered nurse population in 1949, did not enter hospitals in appreciable numbers until the 1960s.[6]

The metamorphosis in the size and complexity of hospital nursing after World War II was dramatic and widespread; it reflected fast-moving change in care of patients as well as shifting responsibilities among nurses, doctors, other caregivers, and families. Strategies to quickly increase the number of nurses, launched in response to perceived post-war nursing shortages, were at the core of many changes in nursing practice.

Shortages of skilled workers plagued professional and occupational groups after the war; nursing was no exception. Post-war mobility, growth in science and technology, and increases in the standard of living shifted public ideas about medical-care accessibility and desirability. Indeed, by the 1960s health protection and hospital care were beginning to be spoken of as the "right" of every citizen. As technological applications of new scientific knowledge offered medical solutions for both acute and chronic illnesses – broad spectrum antibiotics and heart-valve replacement are good examples – the public sought them for themselves and their families.

Hospitals became central players in the successful interplay of a broader societal expectation of the right to health care and a growing emphasis on access to the benefits of science and technology. As community institutions where the achievements of scientific medicine were dispensed to the citizens, hospitals took the responsibility to deliver on the promises of improved morbidity rates and life saving ascribed to the new pharmaceuticals and surgical techniques.

Antibiotic therapy transformed care of pneumonia and other infectious diseases from life-threatening events to short-term illnesses after 1945. The use of sulfa drugs in the 1940s, for example, correlated with a 23 percent decline in death from pneumonia and a 33 percent drop in deaths from meningitis.[7] New surgical advances and technological developments also enabled lives to be saved that previously would have been lost. The combined effects of higher living standards, shifts in the nature and severity of illness, and scientific treatment, significantly reduced morbidity and mortality rates. Life expectancy expanded accordingly. In 1940, the average life expectancy for white males was 62.1 years and 66.6 for white women; this rose to 66.5 and 72.2 respectively by 1950. Figures for black men and women, though lower overall, ranged from 51.5 and 54 in 1940 and from 59.1 and 62 by 1950.[8]

These positive post-war attitudes about the desirability of better access to health care resonated from the interwar period. In 1932, the Committee on the Costs of Medical Care called for organized, coordinated medical care centered around community hospitals, better public health services, insurance or tax support to pay for health care, and upgrading the education of nurses, nurse-midwives and hospital administrators. In spite of opposition from the American Medical Association, especially Morris Fishbein, editor of the *Journal of the American Medical Association*, the report of the Committee on the Cost of Medical Care gave considerable impetus to centralized hospital planning. Moreover, hospital insurance, and later insurance to cover physicians' care, began to spread and make hospitals accessible to more people.

Continuing optimism about improved national health through applied science helped pave the political way for hospital expansion after World War II. The Hospital Survey and Reconstruction Act (Hill Burton), signed by Harry Truman in 1946, provided money for hospital and health-facility development. The Act offered federal assistance to state funding for renovating or building new hospitals and health centers in areas of need, including rural communities and towns with no or dilapidated pre-existing facilities. Moreover, Hill Burton planners projected national hospital bed needs per thousand population as 4.5–5.5 beds for every 1,000 persons in general hospitals, 5 beds per 1,000 persons suffering from mental disorders, 2.5 beds for every 1,000 tuberculosis cases, and 2 beds per 1,000 chronically ill persons. By 1951 there were approximately one million beds in general, mental, tuberculosis, and chronic hospitals across the nation; another 874,000 beds were added in 1952.[9]

Americans' perception of health and hospital care as a basic "right" was further sustained by the post-war boom in employer-provided private hospital insurance. In 1946, a third of the civilian population had some form of private hospital insurance; coverage rose to 50 percent by 1950 and then to 75 percent by 1960.[10] Plans such as Blue Cross were earmarked for middle-class workers and guaranteed their subscribers' access to newly beneficial technology and medical therapeutics found in hospitals.

Hospital expansion, changes in types and amounts of care, shifts in consumer ideology about health, greater individual and national economic surplus, and increasing numbers of older Americans combined to create demand-side strains on the health-care system in general and on nursing in particular. For example, during the late 1950s and early 1960s, creation of intensive care units for physiologically unstable patients required "new nurses" and a subsequent redefinition of nursing's role and responsibilities in hospital settings.[11] As hospitals offered more services and promised better outcomes, costs began to rise. Hospitals sought a larger but cheaper nursing labor force.

The idea of "more is better," rather than "more *and* better," guided most, if not all, nursing-manpower development strategies of the post-war period. "More and better is all right," was Surgeon General Thomas Parran's response to Nursing Chief Lucille Petry of the United States Public Health Service (USPHS) when she laid out her wartime plans to upgrade nursing education, "but [first] it has to be more."[12] Parran's attitude toward nursing was widely shared and would prevail for almost twenty years.

Dominating every discussion of American nursing during the second half of the twentieth century was the debate over the amount, nature and location of nursing education. The growing use of practical nurses and nurse's aides, in conjunction with student nurses and professional nurses, required a new division of nursing labor in hospitals. Dependence on an experience-oriented, apprentice training system for staffing hospitals persisted fifty years longer in nursing than in other fields of work.[13] Failure of the nursing and hospital leadership to directly confront education and hospital staffing problems ensured that nursing would be unready for America's expanded hospital-care initiative after World War II.[14] Expansion of hospitals under the Hill Burton legislation and the spread of voluntary health insurance for medical and hospital care exacerbated an already troubled hospital nursing situation.

Seeking Calm and Competence in the Hospital

"The surface atmosphere of an American hospital is one of calm and competence," wrote author Fred Cook in 1962. "Walk along the corridors on visiting hours and you'll find a nurse behind her desk at the central station, others moving quietly in and out of rooms on their various missions . . . everything looks normal, efficient; all seems under control . . .".[15] In reality, American hospitals after World War II were anything but calm; the situation was virtual chaos. Changes were implemented rapidly with little forethought of how care would be rendered and managed by nursing staffs. Concerned about public acceptance, hospital administrators tried to maintain an aura of calm and competence even as they struggled to find and keep the necessary nurses to staff their hospitals. Shortage of nursing staff was a visible and problematic thorn in the side of hospital administrators and physicians trying to promote scientific and technologic wonders to a consuming American society.

Hospital admissions rose by 25 percent between 1946 and 1952. As the hospital became the center for delivery of scientific and technological know-how and an extension of and substitute for home-based care, patients expected to benefit from state-of-the-art treatments and procedures while being reassured and protected by tender loving care. Nurses were seen as the logical liaisons between science, technology, and community in the institutional "home."[16] A shortage of nurses, therefore, meant more than just too few caregivers. Rather, as described by Margaret Bridgeman in 1953, it was a "critical deficiency in nursing services and a major social problem that impacts hospitals and communities and individual citizens."[17]

Indeed, the post-war shortage of nurses for hospital work drove and informed most of the studies of nursing between 1948 and 1965. Characterized by a certain "eye of the beholder" interpretive style, these studies reveal the participants' ambivalence between economic and non-economic approaches to determining and defining manpower shortages.[18] The studies, most of which were funded by Federal or private non-nursing sources and headed by non-nurse researchers, specified nursing's "problems" and offered prescriptions to nursing for implementation.[19]

Central unresolved questions focused on the appropriate reciprocal relationship between nursing education and nursing work. Could an effective educational strategy be found to serve the interests of nursing candidates and meet hospitals' growing demands for nursing personnel? How could an effective system of higher education prepare sufficient numbers and types of nurses for diversified nursing functions while at the same time maintaining competent and safe care in hospitals?

"Outsider" Prescriptions for Nursing

Three early studies set the stage for research on the "nursing problem" in the 1950s: sociologist Esther Lucile Brown's *Nursing for the Future*; economist Eli Ginzberg's *Program for the Nursing Profession*; and the American Medical Association's *Report on Nursing Problems*. These studies presented a cross-section of medical, hospital, and nursing interests which shared a common goal – to find ways to provide more nurses for American hospitals.

Brown's *Nursing for the Future* emerged from the expanded agenda of the National Nursing Council [for War Services] (NNC). The NNC, organized in 1942, represented nursing and other health interest groups, intended to recruit nurses for military service and increase wartime enrollment in nursing schools. The NNC moved far beyond its initial agenda to involve itself in accreditation, racial integration of nursing, reorganization of nursing's professional organizations, and lobbying for federal funding for nursing education.

Credited by historian and editor Mary Roberts with giving the nursing profession "a dynamic sense of direction and an exciting action program," the Carnegie Foundation-funded "Brown Report" focused specifically on nursing education as a crucial element in the nursing shortage problem.[20] Brown believed there was something fundamentally wrong with a system of education that could not meet the demand for either quantitative or qualitative nursing service. Advised by a committee of nurses, physicians, hospital administrators, academicians, and policy-makers, Brown sought to determine "who should organize, administer, and finance professional schools of nursing," arguing that any decision made should be in the best interests of society and not in "the vested interest for the profession of nursing."[21] From the moment of its publication the report was accepted by nursing and the USPHS leadership as an agenda for nursing reform.

Meanwhile, R. Louise McManus, Chair of Nursing at Teachers College, Columbia University in New York, assembled a committee of experts from a variety of medical and social-science fields. Headed by Columbia University economist Eli Ginzberg, the "Committee on the Function of Nursing" set its sights on the problems of the current and prospective shortages of nursing personnel. "When individuals who have the financial ability to pay for nursing care cannot obtain it; when hospitals with waiting lists are forced to close wards or limit patient admissions . . . when all these circumstances attest to the prevailing shortage [of nurses], its existence can no longer be denied nor its implications neglected."[22]

Again, it was assumed that sensible decision-making about nursing required that individuals outside nursing scrutinize and prescribe solutions to nursing's "problems." The language in these texts speaks of nursing as a commodity, like food and housing, needing improvement as part of the post-war health-care package. The perceived shortage of hospital nurses threatened society's "right to health care"; shortage became the metaphor for a wide array of systemic problems since readily available nursing linked societal expectations of a right to hospital care and institutional claims to scientific and technological expertise.

The American Medical Association's (AMA) Committee on Nursing Problems also sought to solve the perceived crisis in nursing numbers. Concerned that declining numbers of nurses would interfere with the hospital agenda and ultimately physicians' interests, the AMA Committee promoted the idea of recruiting married and retired graduates back into the workforce while simultaneously recruiting new student nurses. At about the same time, the American Nurses Association (ANA) conducted the "Older Nurse Project," emphasizing placement of older nurses back into active nursing service. Actually married and retired graduate nurses returned to the workforce during the war crisis, so the AMA and ANA initiatives were really an attempt to keep these older nurses in the hospitals. "Retired and married nurses," the AMA urged, "should be requested to fill in during the emergency."[23]

Interestingly, this latter recommendation directly conflicted with the post-war message given most other women in the labor force. At the war's end, American women were encouraged to reclaim their domestic domain and "recapture those functions in which they have demonstrated superior capacity . . . the nurturing functions centering around the home."[24] But housework as woman's *raison d'être* tended to be ignored when it came to nurses – at least during periods of shortage. Nursing, as women's work, did not threaten returning veterans' jobs; moreover, nursing services were seen as essential to the greater social good.

How Nurses Saw the "Problem"

Despite the well-known occupational discontent of nurses during this period, none of their concerns figured importantly in the Brown, Ginsberg, or AMA Committee reports.[25] Improvement of working and living conditions and economic security matters took a backseat to the perceived need to increase the numbers of entry-level nurses. Rather than addressing low salaries and long work days to encourage nurses to stay in the field, the committees compiled prospective estimates of the numbers of nurses needed to staff hospitals in the immediate and remote future. The failure to address problems of retention reflected prevailing assumptions about the likely career patterns of nurses, i.e. that they would work only until marriage, and a preference among planners for large numbers of low-cost, entry-level staff nurses rather than more senior and more expensive nurses.

Meanwhile working nurses' explanations of the post-war nursing crisis in hospitals focused on pay and working conditions; complaints of dissatisfaction with pay swept nursing ranks. Lily Mary David's 1947 report to the National Nursing Council listed the top items of job dissatisfaction among nurses: lack of retirement and unemployment security, inadequate quality and quantity of nonprofessional help, undetermined methods of promotion and pay increases, and hourly rates of pay that did not compensate for over-time.[26] Salaries were a constant source of dissension; institutional staff nurses consistently reported being underpaid. In 1947, the average hospital nurse earned $175 per month or $2,100 per year.[27] Fairman, in her analysis of two Philadelphia hospitals, noted that their nurses' average monthly salaries were approximately $40 lower than the amount suggested by the Pennsylvania Nurses Association.[28] Starting salaries for nurses were also consistently lower than salaries for comparable female occupations such as teachers, social workers or librarians.[29] By 1960, nurses earned an annual average of $4,400 compared with $5,410 by elementary school teachers, $4,592 by librarians, and $5,481 by social workers.[30] One mother lamented the wage disparity between her two daughters, one a nurse and the other a teacher, ". . . one daughter [the nurse], after 2 years of college, 2 years in the hospital and another year in college . . . her salary will be $225 per month or $2,700 per year with 2 weeks vacation – the other [the teacher] had 36 months of college with 3 months off each summer . . . her salary is $3,100 for the first year with 3 months vacation."[31]

The nurse's typical scheduled work day was eight hours but her actual average per week was 44 hours. A quarter of the hospital nurses were required to be on call in addition to their normal duty hours. Overtime was unpaid in either case. There were seldom pay differentials for the less desired night shifts. Finally, while nurses averaged two-week vacations and sick leaves, most did not receive either medical-care benefits or insurance.

Trying to Get the Numbers to Work

In 1948 an estimated 299,067 active registered nurses were in the workforce; most of these worked full-time.[32] This was a marginal increase from 284,159 nurses estimated in 1940, in spite of strenuous wartime efforts to increase graduations from nursing schools. The AMA Committee estimated a need for a total of 550,000 nurses by 1960. To accomplish this, 50,000 new nurses would need to graduate each year. Ginzberg disagreed with the AMA figures, saying they did not account for "increased use of practical nurses, decreased use of private duty nurses, increased reliance by the public on the hospital, initiation of pre-payment [insurance] plans, and regional disparity."[33] He projected an annual need for 75,000 new graduates throughout the 1950s.

These contrasting projections suggest that, while early studies came to consensus on shortage, they all worked with unreliable data on the actual numbers of practicing nurses, the factors causing shortage, or factors influencing demand for nurses. Bear in mind that hospital staffs made up of fully trained nurses were still in their infancy when these studies were undertaken; no one knew with any precision how day-to-day nursing care for hospital patients should be changed. Patients in many hospitals still received most of their care from student nurses recruited to the hospital schools in numbers sufficient to meet hospital staffing needs. Many hospital administrators lacked experience of staffing wards with paid care-givers; they had never had to confront the reality of efficient use of nurses since the "schools" always provided the labor force.

In any event supply-side strategies to produce more nurses were implemented in full force. Ginzberg advocated part-time employment for married women and attracting men and non-whites, particularly African Americans, into the nursing profession. In addition, all three committees advocated training "professional" and "nonprofessional" categories of nursing personnel whose work would be differentiated by "class of patient" and "type of function."[34] Using engineering's occupational model, Brown sought to explain the hierarchy of nurse workers. She saw similarities between the work differentiation and occupational preparation of engineers and nurses and thought the parallel with engineering might illuminate an "often bewildering" nursing situation.[35]

Engineers used three basic levels of workers: professional engineers, who provided the intellectual leadership; technicians, who were the operating-level subordinates; and engineering artisans, who provided the bulk of the manual labor.[36] The separation between "school elite" and "shop elite" was a longstanding and intentional pattern of engineering professional practice; school elite or "professionals" advocated the growth of a body of common knowledge and the application of theory to practice, while the shop elite adhered to the value of acquired expertise and an apprenticeship system.[37]

Professional nurses came from the college or hospital-based diploma programs which prepared registered nurses, analogous to the engineers' "school elite"; nonprofessional practical nurses, aides, orderlies and other auxiliary workers were akin to technicians and engineering artisans. But, for nursing, one of the problems with the engineering model would be difficulty classifying collegiate-nurse graduates and diploma graduates in one "school elite" group.

Nonetheless, working out the distinction between professional and nonprofessional nursing practice, agreed Brown and Ginzberg, would guarantee more efficient and effective use of the professional nurse. Lily David reported that "over one fourth of the total hours of institutional nurses were devoted to clerical work, bathing and feeding patients, taking meals to patients, answering lights, taking patients to appointments, and checking linens and supplies."[38] The greater part of professional nurses' days was devoted to preparing and distributing medications, giving treatments, taking temperatures and pulses, and supervising either students or nonprofessional staff.

By redistributing housekeeping and clerical tasks to other workers, it was believed, the professional nurse would be able to concentrate on her "proper task of nursing care and nursing administration."[39] Shifting environmental management from professional nurses to nonprofessionals meant giving up nursing roles and responsibilities traditionally deemed central to nursing practice.[40] But these proposals illustrate the 1950s hope that specific task identification and assembly-line approaches could be used to calculate and control escalating demands for nurses. The system called "team nursing" is the best example of the effort to supplement professional nurses by adding practical nurses and nurse's aides to the work group. The goal was to organize patient care in such a way as to utilize all nursing personnel "in the interest of economy and efficiency."[41]

Efforts to apply scientific management techniques to nursing work were not new. Nurse leaders throughout the twentieth century argued for a division of nursing labor that apportioned nurses' work among different types of nursing personnel, thereby conserving professional nurses' labor.[42] Reverby notes that, "it was precisely a concern with detail, systemizing and proper organization that trained nursing brought to the hospitals."[43]

During the late 1940s and up to the mid-1950s, practical nurses seemed the ultimate solution to the hospital nurse shortage. Deemed capable of safely assuming many of the tasks of professional and student nurses, large numbers of practical nurses, planners believed, offered a solution to nurse-manpower concerns in a relatively affordable and expedient manner. Nurse's aides, popular during the war as voluntary nursing assistants, were also seen as indispensable members of the nursing team who could "render much valuable service as assistants to the professional and practical nurses."[44]

Ginzberg called for a "marked expansion of the numbers of

trained practical nurses with a lesser expansion in the numbers of professional nurses."[45] His bottom-heavy strategy conflicted with the engineering system Brown thought was the right model. According to Brown, professional engineers used lesser-skilled artisans and technicians to maximize their work but simultaneously increased the number of college-prepared engineers to retain balance in practice. Ginzberg's proposal called for the ratio of nonprofessional to professional workers to be "two practical nurses to every one professional nurse."[46]

Brown favored the baccalaureate approach in nursing education to prepare professional nurses but she wrote that the transition from hospital school to college would have to be gradually phased in to avoid a staffing crisis in hospitals. Everyone realized that nurses were essential to the daily workings of the hospital; the training system could not be altered radically because the day-to-day success of hospitals depended on nurses' [read students'] work.

Educating Nurses

In 1959, 1,100 hospital schools of nursing educated almost all the nation's nurses. But hospital leaders increasingly viewed with alarm the rising net costs of nursing education. As their hospitals' nursing needs escalated they began to question the value of student services. William K. Miller, director of the Newport Hospital and a former Chair of the Rhode Island State Committee on Nursing, believed hospitals carried an unfair financial burden as they struggled to produce enough nurses to supply America's nursing workforce. Nurse education costs were often passed on by charging patients higher rates. Miller asserted that "The cost of their education, which has increased sharply and continues to increase, contributes materially to the cost of patient care in those hospitals."[47] Miller spelled out his position using an analysis of the nursing service in his own hospital (tables 1.1 and 1.2).[48]

Reimbursement from insurance for student care of hospital patients helped defray the overall cost of nursing education for both the student and the hospital. Although it documented only one case, the Newport study clarified that the rise in the total number of student service hours was due to increasing numbers of students. Since the number of hours of service *per student* actually decreased, hospitals incurred more expenses to educate each student. Administrators like Miller began to look outside the hospital,

Table 1.1 Comparative summary of net cost of nursing education at Newport Hospital, 1954–1957

Year	1954	1955	1956	1957
Net Cost	$36,657	$51,457	$62,804	$71,747

Table 1.2 Net cost of student service, 1957 – Newport Hospital

Year	1954	1955	1956	1957
Number of Students	52	60	59	78
Total Hours of Student Service	44,233	51,613	52,891	62,288
Hours per Student	851	860	896	799
Value of Student Service	$1.44	$1.20	$1.28	$1.21

seeking a new base for nursing education. Apparently many of Miller's colleagues agreed with his concerns and his calculations; the American Hospital Association supported the 1960s Federal initiatives to finance nursing education.

Beginning in 1952 entirely new schools were created in tax-supported community colleges to prepare registered nurses more rapidly. The number of practical nurses (LPNs) and nurse's aides almost doubled between 1950 and 1962. The quantity of professional nurses also began a significant rise during the 1950s, from 375,000 to 555,000 active nurses by 1962. Growth was influenced by the large number of part-time nurses working and the growing output of two-year associate degree programs (ADN) in community colleges (tables 1.3 and 1.4). The first two-year Associate Degree in Nursing program was established in New York State; by 1963 the idea had spread to 84 programs across the country.[49]

Heterogeneity in Nursing

Relocating nursing education from its traditional base in local hospital schools to mainstream educational institutions, i.e. four-year colleges and two-year associate degree programs in community colleges, acted to segment nursing, creating a caste system with discriminating racial and ethnic undertones. Especially practical

Table 1.3   Numbers of professional and nonprofessional nurses in active practice, 1950–1990

Year	1950	1962	1970	1980	1990
RNs	375,000	550,000	722,000	1.3 mil	2.1 mil
LPNs	137,000	225,000	370,000	549,000	608,000
NAs	220,000	400,000	700,000	850,000	...

Statistics compiled from: US Department of HEW, PHS, *Toward Quality in Nursing: Report of the Surgeon General's Consultant Group on Nursing* (Washington DC: USGPO, 1963); Institute of Medicine, *Nursing and Nursing Education: Public Policies and Private Actions*, p. 53; *Nurse Training Act of 1964: Program Review Report* (Washington DC: USGPO, 1967); US Department of Health and Human Services, *Seventh Report to the President and Congress on the Status of Health Personnel in the United States* (Washington DC: USGPO, 1990).

Table 1.4   Percentage of educational sources of RNs by types of programs of nursing education, 1950–1990

Year	1950	1960	1970	1980	1990
Diploma	83%	84%	52%	19%	8%
Baccalaureate	17%	13%	21%	33%	31%
Associate	...	3%	27%	48%	61%

Data compiled from: US Department of HEW, Nurse Training Act of 1964; US Department of HEW, PHS, *Toward Quality in Nursing: Needs and Goals*; American Nurses' Association, *Facts about Nursing*; National League for Nursing, *Nursing Data Source 1990*, Volume 1: *Trends in Contemporary Nursing Education*, p. 16.

nurses (LPNs), whose numbers nearly doubled from 137,000 in 1950 to 250,000 in 1964, were more likely to be from racial and ethnic minorities than their professional counterparts.[50] Nonwhite practical nurses represented 12.4 percent of the total in 1950 and 17 percent in 1960; professional nurses were still 97 percent white.[51]

Black professional nurses were officially integrated into the American Nurses' Association (ANA) in 1952 when the National Association of Colored Graduates (NACG) voluntarily dissolved. David B. Smith contends that the integration of African Americans into nursing was as much related to nursing's lack of power and hospitals' self-interest as to any altruistic motives in either group. "Medical societies," Smith argued, "were better able to withstand external pressures for integration . . . the more fragile nursing associations were far more responsive to these pressures."[52] He quotes *The*

Nation, which labeled hospital motives for integration as "a case of arriving at the right answer for the wrong reason."[53]

Though black nurses were officially accepted into the traditional white female nursing professional organization, their practices remained concentrated primarily in private duty and public health-practice settings until hospitals were integrated in the late 1960s. Integrated hospitals saw black nurses (who represented less than 4 percent of the total nurse workforce) as a viable option to alleviate the shortage of white female caregivers. African American nurses' acceptance by the public and other caregivers, however, continued fraught with serious challenge and discrimination.[54]

Foreign nurses presented another option to help alleviate the nurse undersupply. Introduced to American hospitals under the 1948 Exchange Visitor Program (EVP), many foreign nurses arrived in the United States as "exchangees" but were used as "employees."[55] Foreign nurses, for the first 15 years of the EVP, were mostly white women from Scandinavia or the British Isles. Their "exchangee" status offered low-paying stipends rather than salaries despite overwhelming evidence that "exchangees" and professional American nurses performed similar functions.[56]

The advantages of using foreign-trained nurses to fill the gaps in the domestic nurse supply were many. First, they were white women from predominantly English-speaking countries, and, despite their accents, they blended into predominantly white hospital nursing staffs rather easily. Second, foreign nurses already trained in their countries of origin did not require education at hospital expense. And last, the status of foreign nurses as exchange visitors enabled hospitals to pay them reduced wages to do the work of nursing. Though the numbers of foreign nurses were relatively small, their use as short-term, temporary workers was consistent with the inexpensive supply-side strategies planners preferred in dealing with increased demand.

Changing Patient Care

Hospitals sought additional ways to reduce operating costs. Having differentiated the nursing workforce, an effort was made to efficiently differentiate hospital patients on the basis of severity of illness using a system called "Progressive Patient Care Model" (PPC). First proposed by the Army in 1951, PPC was later promoted by the nursing leadership in the US Public Health Service as a way to organize facilities, service, and staff around the medical and nursing needs of patients.[57]

Patients were grouped according to their degree of illness and their need for care rather than by the traditional method of diagnosis. There were five basic levels in the progression from most ill to most well: intensive care for the seriously or critically ill; intermediate care for the patient requiring "a moderate amount of care"; self care for the "physically self-sufficient"; long-term care for those needing extensive chronic care; and home care for convalescents and less needy chronically ill persons.[58] Patients' illness determined different levels and amounts of nursing care and, it was hoped, would make more economical use of available nursing staff. The slogan promoting the idea was "the right patient in the right bed at the right time, for the right cost."[59] Progressive patient care, noted Haldeman and Abdellah, "shows promise of helping hospitals with their two most pressing problems: scarcity of trained personnel and continuing improvement of services without unduly increasing costs."[60] When PPC was being promoted the team system of assigning nurses to care for patients was still in vogue but gathering more and more criticism.

The architectural design of each unit was also thought critical to optimal efficiency and care delivery. For instance, intensive care units (ICUs) were designed with "elevated, centrally located nurses' desks to facilitate observation and one or two beds closed off by glazed partitions to provide quiet yet permit visual observation."[61] Self-care units, on the other hand, afforded patients privacy and quiet as they convalesced from surgery or awaited diagnostic testing.

But sorting patients by physiological instability and the intensity of their care needs revealed the difficulties, particularly in early ICUs, of predicting and thus managing care for diverse groups of critically ill patients. Unanticipated patient instability and unpredictable courses of illness created crises and high-pressure nursing-care situations. The question became: was the architectural renovation and centralization of certain nursing staff all that cost-effective and time-efficient, or, in their attempts to modernize were hospitals creating even greater chaos?[62] Ultimately the demands on nurses in intensive care units led them to band together to educate themselves and, during the 1970s, they began to standardize the work of intensive care.[63]

Nursing Administration

Paralleling the changes in nursing education and patient-care strategies was a sharper emphasis on nursing administration and
expansion of the specialty of hospital administration. Well prepared
hospital administrators became particularly important after World
War II as hospital budgets grew and financial control became ever
more critical to hospital survival. The nagging nurse-manpower
problem, added to other burgeoning hospital demands, served as an
impetus for the development of nurse managers. "The next creative
step in the improvement of nursing services," said Herman Finer,
director of the Kellogg Foundation Nursing Service Administration
Research Project, 1950–51, "is better administration."[64]

Directors of nursing services were charged primarily with the task
of "organizing, directing and supervising the nursing service to
insure sufficient and competent nursing care and setting up the
budgeting request and administering the budget appropriation for
the nursing service."[65] To perform these functions it was assumed
that nursing administrators should know the full range of nursing
activities in the hospital. The nurse administrator should "know the
functions she is administering, who ought to be doing them, in what
relationship of teamwork, with what degree of quality, and at what
comparative compensation . . . an intimate, inward acquaintance
with each function is indispensable."[66]

A 1953 survey by the accounting firm of Harris, Kerr, Forester &
Company emphasized the Director of Nurses' financial responsibilities to the hospital. After a thorough analysis they concluded that
nursing administration should initiate their own nursing budgets
and promote economy of nursing services as their primary goal.[67]
Further, the authors encouraged the use of nurse-function studies
as ways to measure nursing efficiency and economy. Herman Finer,
while concurring that time and motion studies were fundamentally
worthwhile, warned that "[they] are liable to become facile
diversions from more difficult, but more important researches in
nursing services, there is a danger of being fascinated by the
obvious."[68]

Women's expertise was not thought to include financial management or institutional planning so directors of nursing who sought
control of the budget and advancement in the hospital hierarchy
found little encouragement. Cultural assumptions about female
subordination to male authority combined with the pervasive view
of nursing's importance to the post-war hospital agenda kept

nursing in a dependent position relative to planning. Hospital administrators and physicians were active participants in nursing planning and decision-making, "fearful of the competition from nurses and unwilling to let a group of women determine their own destiny."[69] Contributing to this picture is the fact that nurses' level of feminist consciousness was at a significantly low point; many nurse supervisors behaved as though incapable of independent thought without hospital administrator or physician direction.

Developments in nursing administration during this period emphasized the internal domestic management of nurses' work. Final decisions about appropriate nurse staffing to minister to the numbers and types of patients admitted to the hospital was usually outside of the responsibility of nursing managers. These crucial decisions remained the province of senior hospital administrators who were neither physicians or nurses.

National Nursing Organizations

Although nursing's national professional organizations dated from the turn of the twentieth century, they were best described as a loose coalition of several overlapping interest groups. A member of the American Nurses' Association, for example, might belong to the government nursing section, the private duty section, the men's nursing section, the administrators of nursing service section, or the industrial nursing section. The National League for Nursing Education (NLNE) siphoned off nurse educators. When national nursing organizations reorganized in 1952, the NLNE became the National League for Nursing (NLN). Until the 1952 reorganization, the National Association of Colored Graduate Nurses represented the voices of nonwhite nurses, who were often barred from entry into white professional organizations. Another coalition were visiting nurses and public health nurses, who, until 1952, looked to the National Organization of Public Health Nursing (NOPHN) for leadership. Thus, while all the various organizations were active and invested energy in such areas as licensing laws, standards of nursing education, and socioeconomic issues, long-term division among nurses prevented the formation of "one strong voice."

Thus, the pre-World War II nursing leadership was fragmented and the larger body of nurses lacked professional cohesion. This organizational disarray of nursing contributed in large part to the tension between nursing agendas and those of various other interest groups. Earlier professionalizing efforts by nurse leaders were often vain attempts by the minority to convince the mass of individual nurses of the need to control their practice. To make matters more difficult, physicians, hospital administrators, and sometimes nurses themselves continued to resist nursing's efforts to professionalize and gain control of its educational system.[70]

After the war, however, nurses began to be labeled "professional" or "nonprofessional" by the very people who had previously opposed nursing professionalization. Hospitals newly staffed with "professional nurses" and their helpers promised expert nursing care. It was the definition of "expert," however, that would prove to be elusive.[71] What was clear was that all of nursing was profoundly affected by the obligation to ensure continuity of both time, i.e. 24 hours and 7 days a week, and place, i.e. the hospital, for patient care.[72] Because professional nurses did not have a monopoly on the work they did, practical nurses with one year of training and nurse's aides, who were trained on the job, were used interchangeably with nurses who held professional licenses. The lines between professional nurses, licensed practical nurses and nursing assistants were quite elastic, resulting in jurisdictional disputes.[73] The ambiguous role of the practical nurse, who earned only 75 percent of the professional nurses' salary but often did the same work, attracted comment. One author wryly noted, "Within many hospitals the practical nurse is not allowed to chart or give medications from 7 a.m. through 3 p.m., but by some feat of alchemy, becomes steadily more competent with the passing hours, so that by 11 p.m. she is carrying the entire nursing service on a ward."[74]

Registered nurses complained bitterly about competition from practical nurses in their professional journals. Faced with the rising numbers of nonprofessionals, many professional nurses argued that the different levels of nurses should be set apart, if not by job functions, then at least by physical appearances or differential titling.

> I believe the public is still being fooled when the practical nurse wears the same uniform as the professional nurse . . . there should be a way patients could distinguish the LPN from the RN at a glance.

> . . . nurses worry about the practical nurse, the bedside nurse, the R.N., and the professional nurse . . . professional nurses should be differentiated from "nurses" by changing her title.[75]

Hospitals that could pay less for labor and still get the job done had an incentive to increase numbers of auxiliary personnel.

Theoretically, by substituting lesser-skilled laborers for workers with higher relative skills, salary savings could be realized while higher quality work could be squeezed from professionally motivated nurses. But low salaries contributed to high turnover among professional nurses. Fairman notes that, "neither the solution nor the problem was simply one of numbers; pouring personnel into the system could not stop the flow out of the system . . . in 1955, the national turnover rate for professional nurses stood at 67 percent, compared to 40 percent for female factory workers."[76] Hospitals, nevertheless, continued for some time to fill the gaps with lesser-skilled workers while capping wages on professional nurses' salaries. The end result was "large proportions of inexperienced nurses [caring for] a growing number of unstable patients."[77]

Trying to Set National Practice Standards

While the nursing leadership failed to control the development and employment of other workers, they kept trying to clarify the work of nursing and establish clear boundaries around the various nursing positions. To accomplish this agenda, the ANA sponsored a series of studies of nursing functions. These studies tried to define nurses' work and determine how nurses' time was distributed among specific, named activities. Primarily fact-finding, the studies were launched in various types of hospitals throughout the country. The ANA Board of Directors listed their general objectives:

1 To determine the functions and relationships of institutional nursing personnel of all types – professional nurses, practical nurses, and auxiliary workers – in order to improve nursing care and utilize nursing personnel most economically and effectively.
2 To determine the proportion of nursing time provided by each group in various situations.
3 To develop techniques for achieving the first two objectives which could be applied to all types of hospitals, and so obtain a national picture.[78]

The ANA Technical Committee drew up a Master Plan for the nursing function studies to be carried out by state and local groups or by contracted research organizations affiliated with state nursing associations. The ANA anticipated that the research "pieces," collected state-to-state and institution-to-institution would fit into an overall pattern for analysis. "How are these much multiplied tasks, calling for varying degrees of intelligence and technical sophistication and ranging from bed bath to lumbar puncture, divided among the large and heterogeneous company of women who are all called 'nurses'?"[79] The ANA hoped this information would enable it to create specific methods to implement changes in practice.

Hughes et al. collated many of the ANA studies in their book *Twenty Thousand Nurses Tell their Story*, noting some general trends and conditions. Despite considerable differences between hospitals, numbers of available staff, types of patients, and methods of data collection (though all studies did use timed functions as the core variable), the general consensus was that, "the care of the person, the bedside, or 'touch' tasks – is now largely in the hands of auxiliary nurses . . . it is as though education were separating the nurse from her patient."[80]

In 1954, Abdellah and Levine discovered that professional nursing staff spent less time with direct patient care than did any other nursing staff.[81] Ford and Stephenson, in their study of three Alabama hospitals, reported that the only tasks differentiating registered nurses from licensed practical nurses and aides were administering intravenous medications and blood transfusions. All other functions varied across the three nursing groups, with RN and LPN activities being the most interchangeable.[82] Others noted the extraordinary amounts of time professional nurses spent on clerical and administrative activities compared with direct patient care.[83] The duties of the Head Nurse best characterized the paperwork functions of RNs. After helping care for patients, the Head Nurse "still had her charts, reports, requisitions and a million-and-one bits of paper work which she is not supposed to delegate, to attend to."[84] Genevieve Meyer wrote that "the continuing change in nursing functions has meant an increase in supervisory duties for the [professional] nurse, while the practical nurse and the aide, whom the nurse supervises, have assumed many direct patient care tasks which used to belong to the nurse."[85]

One of the main problems with the nurse-function studies was identifying "direct patient care" or differentiating "non-nursing" from "nursing" skills. In one of the first studies undertaken under the ANA's Program of Studies of Nursing Functions, Phoebe Gordon tried to attach meaning to these terms.[86] But twenty or more of these studies of nursing functions reveal little consistency of interpretation among researchers using these key terms.

Donald Stewart, who assessed four Arkansas hospitals and

analyzed "17,145.5 minutes observed among 36 RNs," for example, concluded that the function of the general duty nurse was determined by three major variables: the structure of the hospital nursing service, the nurse's place in the hospital infrastructure, and the individual characteristics of the nurse.[87] Structure of the hospital nursing service included hospital size, the type of control of nursing service, the size of the professional nursing staff, and the numbers and types of auxiliary nursing personnel. Hours of work, types of services provided, numbers of patients cared for and actual patient conditions determined nurses' place in the infrastructure. Education, experience, and motivation defined the individual characteristics of the nurse.

Stewart made a key observation relative to the ANA's nursing-function studies. He found the definition of nursing functions non-generalizable on the basis of results from individual hospitals. Surveys of 40 hospitals in California could not inform nursing needs in Michigan any more than Kansas findings would generalize to Washington. Each state and each institution had its own unique hospital culture, organization, and structure, and each defined the status and role of nursing on the basis of its own set of circumstances.[88]

Since nurses' varying functions depended on local factors, study results were misleading or inconclusive when aggregated. Measuring nurses' work by collating timed activities did not capture the multitude of non-quantifiable influences on nurses' changing caregiving responsibilities. The studies did not account for variations among hospital size, patient illness, staffing needs, shifts worked, insurance mechanisms, or a host of other variables. They did not consider the actual work of caring as a manifestation of substitution for family care at home, i.e. "women's work."

The caring work of nursing proved difficult, actually impossible, to measure. It eluded rational, quantitative analysis. Herman Finer, in particular, criticized time and motion studies. He argued that quality nursing care is "nonmeasurable" and that "the nursing profession must face the fact that . . . [its works are] not susceptible of precise or statistical measurement and statement."[89] Nevertheless, most post-war responses to nursing shortages were based on and limited by simple and measurable economic assumptions.[90]

Years of Rapid Growth and Change

> Even the sturdiest character may quail before the pressures of work and responsibility nurses often face in hospitals today, and turnover has been high, making the work load heavier for those staff members remaining on the job. New forms of treatment, early ambulation, short hospital stays, and changing concepts of hospital responsibility for total health care have multiplied the nursing tasks per patient day and increased their complexity.[91]

A combination of post-war social, cultural, political, and economic influences determined and shaped the changes in nursing practice in the 1950s. Americans, fresh from war, and experiencing an economic strength previously unknown, desired the best health care money could buy. Nursing was part of the health-care package. Scientific and technological developments accentuated societal expectation for rights to health care. As scientific treatment dominated hospital settings, nurses became even more valuable to the institution as technicians and caretakers. Their presence was necessary to the security of the hospital as much as to the security of the nation. In many ways, the community hospital was a microcosm of post-war America. It was a place of restoration to health as the country restored itself to peace and prosperity. High expectations of hospital nurses, however, were not yet accompanied by changes in education or status.

Nurses followed the patients; as care became centralized in hospitals, nursing employment in hospitals increased. But cultural influences and the beliefs and values of society were faithfully reflected in hospitals, making the women staff nurses second-class citizens in growing and more complex systems that tended to assign effective power to men. As women, nurses' patterns of employment were susceptible to the authority of men – both physicians and a growing cadre of male hospital administrators.[92] Had nursing been a profession mostly made up of men, it is less likely that interested "outsiders" would have felt compelled or been able to intervene and make decisions about its practice, education, and manpower needs. Most likely it would also have been harder to steadfastly ignore complaints about working conditions and pay.

Political influences governed the allocation, transference and sharing of power in local hospitals; as nursing's principal employers they exerted virtual monopsonistic power over nurses' incomes. Monopsony is the market condition that exists when there is only one buyer for goods or services. With the war over and the general decline of private duty nursing, nurses' major independent employment option gradually disappeared. Nurses became ever more reliant on hospitals for their livelihoods and the majority of nursing schools were still housed and financed by hospitals. It became common practice, where there was more than one hospital in a community, for administrators to agree on salaries, thus avoiding competition.

Another, more elusive change in the years after World War II was the shift in the meaning of the word "nurse." Prior to the war, "nurse" was assumed to mean either a student apprentice or a trained graduate. Students were the mainstay nursing workforce of pre-war hospitals; graduate nurses practiced in private homes upon graduation. The war and the subsequent boom in hospital care, insurance incentives, and the "right to care" ideology – with their pressures for more nurses – forged a hierarchical structure in nursing. After the war a "nurse" could be a student, graduate or practical nurse, an aide, or an orderly. Consequently, the definition of "nurses' work" became increasingly blurred.

Post-war studies of nursing sought to solve the perceived nursing shortage with readily implemented, low-cost solutions. In doing so, they dealt with the immediate crisis – while disregarding the long-term implications for nursing or patient care. In this sense nursing expansionism mirrored hospital expansionism in the lack of debate about the underlying assumptions on which expansion was based. Operating under "more is better" thinking, planners chose supply-side strategies to solve poorly defined "crises." Practical nurses and other nonprofessional nursing staff replaced the unpaid student labor that was gradually curtailed in the 1950s and 1960s. Although originally conceived as temporary solutions these workers remained, further dividing nursing by race, class, and education. Hospital segmentation of nursing, therefore, was both a politically expedient and an economically determined strategy.

The ANA's attempt to establish a national picture of nursing by combining local and state-wide studies of nursing functions failed. The studies only succeeded in demonstrating that nursing practices in particular institutions reflected local community conditions. Rather than developing an influential nationwide analysis of nursing as had been hoped, the ANA studies revealed a confusing picture of individualistic, even idiosyncratic practices in individual hospitals.

Unlike many other occupations in short supply during the 1950s, nursing did not gain in the struggle for income and status. For example, in 1947, the average hospital nurse earned $175 monthly or around $2,100 annually.[93] Fifteen years later, though nurses' annual income had more than doubled to $4,400, it had not kept pace with other comparable women's professions: elementary school teachers, librarians, and social workers, who earned $5,310, $4,592, and $5,481 respectively.[94] Hospitals' centrality in medical care and their economic interests outweighed nursing's appeal for equity and advancement. Because nurses could not articulate their worth and failed to define their work as a monopoly to either themselves, hospitals, or physicians, they found themselves underpaid and inexpensively substituted for by practical nurses, nurse's aides, and other assistive personnel.

The addition of this roster of assistive nursing personnel forced staff nurses into administrative and supervisory roles. In 1960, Genevieve Meyer noted the reverberating effect of increasing technical demands on nurses, arguing that the technical role was growing into an administrative–technical role as professional nurses were forced to supervise practical nurses and nurse's assistants.[95] But little attention was paid to significant changes in medical practice and the likely impact of those changes on nurses' work during this period.[96]

The "more is better" ideology ensured enough hospital workers to manage the lightning-paced changes in science-based diagnosis and treatment. It allowed women who were turned away from "men's work" an avenue for noncompetitive job entry and enabled

Table 1.5   Active health manpower per 100,000 population, 1950–1986

Year	1950	1960	1970	1980	1986
MDs	144	144	158	190	218
RNs	246	279	342	560	660

Source: Department HEW, *Hearing of the Committee on Appropriations* (1971); National Center for Health Statistics, *Statistical Abstract of the United States – 1972*, p. 5; US Health and Human Services, PHS, *Health of the United States, 1988* (DHHS Pub. No. 89-1232, 1988).

nonwhite and lower-class women access to nursing. Between 1950 and 1967 numbers of registered nurses rose by 67 percent, licensed practical nurses by 134 percent, and nursing aides/assistants by 244 percent.[97] Numbers of physicians, on the other hand, rose much more slowly in this period.[98] About 16,000 nurses practiced in the public mental-health system with its more than 700,000 beds; 64,000 (10 percent of the total) nurses were still practicing as private duty nurses.[99] (See table 1.5.)

Although post-war initiatives focused on the supply of nurses, exhortations to improve the quality of nursing practice began to gain ground. The very title of the 1963 federal government report *Toward Quality in Nursing* revealed increasing worry both within and outside nursing about the abilities of nurses in the workforce.

2

Reorganizing Care, 1960–1980

The Sixties and Seventies

Better access created by the continued expansion of Blue Cross and Blue Shield as well as other hospital insurance faced hospitals with growing demand for beds, a larger proportion of aged persons occupying those beds, and rising costs (twice the inflation of other prices in 1966). Calls for more nurses escalated as did new efforts to improve hospital nursing care. Throughout the 1960s some still hoped that the Progressive Patient Care (PPC) idea could increase efficiency and raise productivity in hospital nursing. The PPC concept stratified the amount of care according to acuity of patient care needs. Implementation of PPC, however, meant that patients would be moved from unit to unit depending on the intensity or amount of nursing care they needed. As it turned out, the original five-level PPC plan proved unwieldy to implement and financially problematic. The intensive nursing care part of the concept worked and spread rapidly so that, by 1969, more than half of all community hospitals boasted some kind of intensive nursing care unit.

The Medicare and Medicaid legislation of 1965, entitling persons over 65 and the poor to physician, hospital, and other medical services, immediately and dramatically increased pressure on both hospitals and nurses.[100] At about the same time, the so-called "Primary Health Care" movement responded to Americans' demand for access to low-cost ambulatory health services. With help from federal dollars, neighborhood health centers, early disease-detection units, and other treatment and prevention efforts tried to counteract and reduce the growing dependence on hospitals. Reducing length of stay for hospitalized patients coupled with insistence that home-care agencies reorient some of their programs to serve the chronically ill were two ways planners hoped to control exploding hospital costs. Both voluntary visiting nurse associations and public-health nursing departments were encouraged to devote more resources to chronically ill and elderly patient care in the home. Limited insurance or other dollars committed to support non-hospital-based health-care services inhibited the impact of all these ambulatory or home-based care ideas.

For nurses in hospitals, the late sixties demanded not only more caregivers, but better-trained people to cover the 24-hour day as the acutely ill proportion of patients rose and the average stay in the hospital grew shorter. Changes in diagnostic and therapeutic management of certain illnesses led to fewer admissions for diagnosis and fewer convalescent patients occupying hospital beds.[101] Hospitals renovated patient care space again in the early 1970s, this time to build more efficient intensive care units. The ratio of nurses to patients rose in intensive care units and the relative number of staff nurses also increased. At the same time, the concept of primary nursing for in-patient care began to spread. This system, which partially replaced team nursing, called for each hospital patient to have an assigned "primary" nurse who would be responsible for his/her care throughout the hospitalization.

Patients in the nation's ever more numerous nursing homes increasingly resembled those who had occupied the community hospitals of the 1950s [the chronically ill elderly] but, because of low pay and poor working conditions, only a few nurses followed these patients into long-term care settings. Hospitals continued to employ the majority of nurses even as nurses were also sought to staff the new primary health-care clinics and home-care agencies.

Specialization in nursing, especially in psychiatric mental-health, intensive care, nurse-midwifery, nurse practitioner practice in ambulatory care and illness-specific practice such as oncology and nephrology nursing, expanded quickly in an ad hoc, segmented fashion in the late 1960s and early 1970s. Central to many changes in this period was renegotiation of the patient care responsibilities of physicians and nurses both in and out of hospitals. Both disciplines gradually adapted to the changing scientific, technological, fiscal and social context in which they found themselves.

Nurses' education continued to relocate from hospital-owned schools to tax-based community-college programs and to private and public baccalaureate programs in colleges and universities. After 1965, federal dollars for nursing education (eventually totaling $1.6 billion) supported expansion of basic programs and higher education at the master's and doctoral level.

Graduates of associate degree programs in community colleges proliferated during the latter part of this period. In some regions these nurses began to experience problems in advancing their careers. Their basic education did not adequately equip them for the ever more complex demands of hospital nursing. The stratification and poor fit of nursing education and nursing practice required nurses to constantly re-train; one out of every ten nurses engaged in formal re-training. The debate about the long-run costs of re-training nurses who gain entry to the profession via brief introductory education versus investing in more elaborate (baccalaureate or higher) introductory education began in the sixties and continues to the present.[102]

"Unusual and Uncustomary" – Nursing Practice after 1965

In 1966, Frances Reiter, an influential nursing leader from New York City, sharply criticized the kind of nursing care provided by what she called a "pyramid of personnel." As noted earlier, some critics estimated that professional nurses gave only about 30 percent of the patient care in 1950s hospitals. A government-sponsored study in 1954 reported that nursing time with patients totaled less than one hour per day. For each patient, they calculated that registered nurses spent 12 minutes, nursing students 18 minutes and licensed practical nurses 18 minutes actually in direct contact in any one day.[103]

Reiter argued that it was almost impossible for hospital patients to obtain personal professional nursing care at their bedside since the "team nursing" system merely spread a limited amount of available nursing service to all patients. The nursing team leader, according to Reiter, was concerned with the *amount* of care each patient got, no matter the quality. Reiter argued vehemently for a better educated, more capable nurse who would be concerned with the *kind* of care patients in hospitals would get.

Nurses seemed to share Reiter's frustration with the hospital work environment for, in spite of the rising numbers of nurses and their assistants, and in spite of the fact that about 70 percent of nurses were working at nursing, hospitals continued to report position vacancies for registered nurses. The national turnover rate for registered nurses in hospitals remained high – 67 percent compared with 40 percent for factory workers.

In 1963 *Toward Quality in Nursing* recommended hospital staffing patterns using 50 percent RNs, 30 percent LPNs and 20 percent aides, but those tracking hospital labor in the mid-1960s thought hospitals actually sought out and employed higher ratios of registered nurses whenever they could get them. The straightforward focus on numbers of caretakers began to shift as many began to worry more about problems of patient safety and satisfaction with care.[104] Doris Schwartz, one of post-war nursing's most thoughtful and imaginative clinical innovators, commented on the problem before the World Health Organization (WHO) Expert Committee on Nursing in 1966. "In the years since the close of World War 2," she wrote, "American nursing has changed so rapidly that in many ways it has left us *knowing* better than we *do* . . . the speed of certain kinds of technological change, and the distribution of the consumers of topnotch health care, has left us *doing* without really knowing how. In the words of the Gilbert and Sullivan operetta: 'Here's a pretty mess'."[105]

In 1967 the National Advisory Commission on Health Manpower (NAC) recommended that "nursing be made a more attractive profession by such measures as appropriate utilization of nursing skills, increased levels of professional responsibilities, improved salaries, more flexible hours for married women, and better retirement provisions."[106] The Commission characterized American health care as in "crisis." Heralding the changed thinking of the times, it was not, they argued, due simply to the low number of nurses; instead they cited problems of poor distribution and varying quality of nursing services.

As would prove true of future public panels, the Commission could not commit itself to a higher standard of entry-level education for nurses because it feared diminishing the supply of hospital nurses.[107] The whole matter of supply of nurses and quality of nursing care rested on value judgments of people with very different perspectives. The concept of need [for nurses] is based on professional standards, which, of course, change over time and often defy quantifying. The concept of demand is economic – "the volume of labor an employer is willing to purchase at a given wage level."[108] Purchasers focused on the costs of increasing numbers of fully prepared nurses while professionals focused on optimal staffing patterns to ensure high quality patient care. So, although the National Advisory Commission did emphasize what came to be called "the qualitative nursing shortage" it did not convert its concern into a logical, though painful conclusion, i.e., calling for more expensive, better trained nurses.

The nursing education system of the 1960s was guaranteed to produce an oversupply of under-prepared nurses unable to fully assume expanding responsibilities in hospitals and unlikely to be appropriately compensated. There was nothing new about this problem. May Ayres Burgess, an economist who studied nursing and nursing education in the late 1920s and early 1930s, repeatedly decried the persisting inconsistency between patterns of nursing education and the nurse labor supply in her several articles and books.[109]

The Commission did call for university nursing schools to assume "responsibility for nursing services" – an idea quite new at the time.[110] This theme of "unification" of university nursing programs with teaching hospitals where nurses could obtain their clinical education would gain credence during the 1970s.

Relationships between Nurses and Physicians

Odin Anderson, writing from the University of Chicago's Center for Health Administrative Studies in the 1960s, saw the problem of quality in hospital nursing somewhat differently. He noted the gap between the discretionary authority and judgment required of the hospital nurse and [her] usual preparation for, and permission to openly execute, those responsibilities. Noting that the physician was infrequently present in the hospital, Anderson nicely captured the ambiguity of the 1960s hospital nurses' situation. The absent physician was held accountable for all clinical/patient-care decisions even though the nurse was the one who was physically present.[111] Anderson urged upgrading of the nurse's responsibility and authority in institutional settings to resolve this unworkable situation.

Anderson's point was inadvertently demonstrated by the language of an earlier study called "Quality of Nursing Care – A Report of a Field-Study to Establish Criteria." Conducted between 1950 and 1954 by the same Frances Reiter mentioned earlier and her colleague Marguerite Kakosh, it attempted to define nursing care by clarifying independent nursing actions versus actions ordered by physicians. The two researchers outlined myriad details of direct, personal care, which they labeled as the independent work of the nurse. However, they acknowledged that the nurse would only function independently in providing nutrition, sleep, elimination, skin care, exercise, and teaching to patients, for example, "unless [these items of care were] prescribed by the physician."[112] It seems evident that the problem nagging nurses in the 1960s was not only that they might be ill prepared for what they faced each day at work but that they couldn't be sure what part of nursing care was theirs to determine or if all was the doctor's responsibility.

In a 1966 commentary on nursing's ambiguous situation, nursing school dean Laurie M. Gunter argued that the field was "declining in value and . . . heading toward obsolescence." Before World War II, she noted, nursing had about as many useful interventions to offer the patient as medicine. Sponging patients to reduce fever, careful feeding, bathing and personal care – all offered as much, or more, help as the pre-war physician's limited pharmacological and therapeutic regimens.

But, with the advent of antibiotics and other therapies, the armamentarium of the physician quickly gained clinical ascendancy and value over nursing care. The hospital patient of the 1960s seldom even knew who his nurse was, although he always knew his doctor. Dean Laurie Gunter worried about the intensive-care movement, believing that it focused nursing energy on diagnosis and therapy rather than promoting the comfort and well-being of patients. As did many nurses, she worried about splitting the so-called professional work of supporting and teaching patients away from "technical" personal care and medical assistant work and wondered how such an artificial split could ever be applied in practice.

Gunter wanted university schools of nursing to link up with hospitals to ensure that higher education for nurses would be firmly grounded in clinical work. Finally, she called for better definition of specialty practice in nursing – urging that nursing specialization be grounded in a sound scientific base. Although Gunter's forecast of nursing's imminent demise proved to be overly gloomy, she proved prescient in many of her predictions. Especially foresighted was her recognition that nursing would soon have to prepare master's-level nurse specialists to cope with the explosive scientific and technological changes in health care.[113]

The Day-to-Day Work of the Hospital Nurse

For staff nurses, work on the typical 1960s hospital unit was difficult and demanding. Traditionally, patients were admitted to rooms
according to their sex, diagnosis, admitting physician, and ability
to pay. Patients were segregated on different units according to
whether they had insurance, were able to pay cash, or were relying
on charity. Clustered together regardless of different nursing needs
in terms of intensity, some patients were capable of self care or
needed intermediate care, others needed post-operative observation, and some needed constant nursing observation and care. If a
patient was critically ill, the family would try to hire a private duty
nurse if they could find and afford one.[114] Often, however, requests
for private duty nurses went unfulfilled so extra nursing care paid
for by the family was an unrealistic option.

Most of the time the staff "made do." Care was still given by
"teams" of nurses and assistants using the "team nursing" method
of patient-care assignment introduced in the early 1950s. The work
of patient care was divided into specific tasks by the team leader,
who was usually a registered nurse; a student or graduate nurse gave
medications, and various nursing assistants and licensed practical
nurses (LPNs) did the rest. There might be 45 to 60 patients per unit;
these were grouped into two or three clusters of 15 to 20 per team.
One or two graduate nurses, three or four students and one or two
LPNs or nursing assistants tended to each group of patients. As
Frances Reiter and other critics of the 1960s said, the nursing team
leader often simply divided up the work and hoped for the best.

Nurses felt they could not keep pace with the problems of their
sickest patients. One nurse remembers those years.

> I remember having a patient on an Aramine drip. He was just across
> from the nurses' station, supposedly so I could keep a close eye on
> him. But I also had 15 or 20 other patients with varying degrees of
> illness on my floor. I would run in to take a blood pressure; if it was
> all right, I would breathe a sigh of relief and go on to my other
> patients. When the drip needed titrating, I would speed it up or slow
> it down a bit [with a roller clamp] and hope for the best.[115]

These nurses felt guilty when their patients got into trouble and
frustrated when they repeatedly faced these hectic conditions.
Physicians also were alarmed by the unpredictable quality and availability of nursing care in hospitals.

Enhancing the ability of nurses to assume a new and different level of authority began to be recognized as the key to better patient survival in hospitals. Nurses and physicians who were closest to patient care rather quickly realized that close collaboration and shared decision-making were crucial to success in patient care. For the most unstable patients, at least those whose conditions seemed to promise recovery if carefully treated, the intensive care units promised a better chance of survival.

In fact, the tension and absurdity of traditional restrictions on nursing practice, i.e. waiting for physicians' orders before intervening, became glaringly evident in the emerging intensive care units which were part of the Progressive Patient Care idea of the late 1950s.[116] In poorly staffed hospitals nurses increasingly confronted desperately ill and dying patients whose medical needs exceeded their knowledge and authority. Left on their own by senior physicians and house officers who either could not come or could not answer their clinical questions, these nurses realized their need for more clinical knowledge about how the heart works, about body chemistry, and about the feasibility and techniques of sustaining life in the face of failing circulation and respiration.

Rose Laub Coser's analysis of the authority relations between hospital medical interns and nurses suggested that doctors and nurses maintained their "ideology of patient centeredness" as a consensual basis from which to operate in actual practice.[117] Even though nurses and physicians could not withdraw from the paradoxical status relationship in which they found themselves, they cooperated around patient care.

In 1967 Leonard Stein wrote the most captivating analysis of the tense, compromised working relationship between nurses and physicians in his popular article "The Doctor–Nurse Game."[118] Stein outlined the rules of the "game." Nurses must be bold, show initiative, and be responsible for making timely and important recommendations, while at the same time appearing passive, so that their recommendations would seem to be initiated by the physician. The important thing in the game was to avoid open disagreement and to maintain the traditional, hierarchical relationship between doctors and nurses. Stein's article, along with others by sociologists, physicians and economists, signaled increasing restiveness among physicians and nurses with their traditional but anomalous working relationship.[119]

Inventing Intensive Care

Nurses responsible for critically ill patients got information about their patients and support for their decisions from physician allies, who were usually cardiologists and/or surgeons. Nurses also banded together to learn what they needed to know from each other. In a late twentieth-century variation on the Promethean myth, they sought to steal the fire of knowledge from Olympus and give it to the "people," intending to transfer previously restricted medical knowledge to themselves.[120] As they look back on those days, critical-care nurses repeatedly phrase their drive to learn in personal and urgent terms – "if you [didn't] know what there [was] to know . . . you always [thought] it is your fault [if something went wrong]."[121]

In the developing field of intensive and "coronary" care, nurses learned on the job, through courses offered by physicians, or from salesmen for manufacturers promoting diagnostic equipment. As one pioneering nurse from Springdale, Arkansas, put it, "doctors and nurses trained each other, and, after a year or so, the nurses were smarter than the doctors."[122] But isolated, unstandardized, and poorly supported local efforts were inadequate in the face of proliferating intensive-care demands in America's general hospitals. As noted earlier, by 1969 more than 50 percent of general hospitals claimed some sort of intensive care unit.[123]

Hospitalized patients died of hypovolemic shock, airway obstruction and respiratory failure, wound hemorrhage, toxicity from infection, starvation and dehydration due to gastrointestinal obstruction [often the result of cancer] and a host of other immediate causes. Of these causes of death the ones most readily detected by round-the-clock nursing vigilance were shock, airway obstruction, infection, and wound hemorrhage.

Cardiac and other chronic disease had pushed infectious diseases off the chart as the leading cause of American death and morbidity much earlier in the century. As one consequence, post-war hospitals admitted large numbers of patients suffering from various manifestations of heart disease. Estimates of the short-term mortality from acute myocardial infarction ranged from 30 percent to 40 percent with nearly half dying from arrhythmias. In the late 1950s patients with chest surgery, those who underwent the then-novel heart-valve replacement procedures, and others, risked post-operative complications ranging from respiratory failure and shock to wound infections or wound drainage problems.

Importantly, these gravely ill patients were newly judged to be "savable." New expectations about the possibility of surviving major physiological assaults of various kinds changed the behavior of both health professionals and the public with regard to care in myocardial infarction and major chest and heart surgery. The management of major casualties during World War II and the Korean conflict led to a new American optimism about emergency and intensive care for civilians. Thus, patients and their families, as well as their doctors and nurses, began to share a different and much more expansive idea of routine treatment in the face of life threatening, devastating illness.[124]

Gravely ill patients overwhelmed the recovery room and private nursing-care systems which preceded the intensive care units. Ultimately, these surgical and cardiac patients, later joined by patients whose lives were prolonged by kidney dialysis, constituted a larger and larger sub-population of hospital patients whose demanding care requirements accentuated the crisis in nursing availability, knowledge and authority. Delay in recognizing the knowledge needs of nurses and the cumulative impact of the care requirements of these acutely ill patients forced "grass-roots" solutions.

Since the majority of hospital nurses had graduated from hospital-based diploma programs their base knowledge of physiology, pathophysiology, and pharmacology was usually at an introductory level. They had been told, and were expected to be able, to rely on physician knowledge to manage clinical problems beyond their own preparation or experience. Nurses' personal expertise developed on the job, especially in rapidly changing areas of practice such as cardiac and post-operative nursing. But only some of the nurses' physician colleagues followed the new trends in cardiology and fewer still were familiar with advances in respiratory support.

This is not surprising; closed chest massage was introduced in 1960, direct-current cardiac defibrillation in 1962, and the early coronary care units at Toronto, Kansas City and Philadelphia were not discussed in the literature until 1962. Older physician generalists were often unfamiliar or uncomfortable with these innovations and did not themselves have easy access to updates on new clinical knowledge or therapeutic entities.

Nurses and their physician specialist allies, confronting daily crises caused by rising acuity among their patients, turned to the precedent of the recovery room. The post-operative recovery room, first introduced just before and during World War II, was the product of a long and difficult management struggle in hospitals. Usually located close to the operating suite, the recovery room provided transitional after-care to patients undergoing major surgery. Each person was closely monitored until he or she recovered consciousness. The idea of the recovery room signaled a new kind of hospital nursing. Hospitals gradually hired a core of full-time graduate nurses to replace private duty nurses formerly selected and paid for by the patients.[125]

But it still took about ten years, from 1962 to the early seventies, to choose and develop the intensive-care approach to some of the quality problems in hospital nursing – improving safety, observing, and intervening in a timely manner. For the most physiologically unstable patients at least, these perennial care issues began to be addressed by nurses who, with support from medical specialists, expanded the boundaries of their practice.

Primary Nursing

Proposals to improve the quality of nursing care for other hospital patients also attracted support in the late 1960s. Marie Manthey's idea to connect a specific hospital nurse, the "primary" nurse, to each patient was launched in 1968.[126] "Primary Nursing" intended that each patient would have a personal professional nurse throughout each hospitalization; this plan responded to Frances Reiter's complaint about team nursing. That is, the relationship between the nurse and the patient under the primary nursing system superseded the "team" approach, which related the nurse to the aggregated work on the patient care unit. In team nursing the nurse and team cared for patients who happened to be in a specific set of rooms. In primary nursing the nurse and patient were associated as individuals, thus, theoretically at least, combating the depersonalization of a bureaucratic system of delivering nursing care.[127]

In 1978, Myrtle Aydelotte, a respected observer of nursing administration, estimated that primary nursing required a hospital nursing staff of 50 to 56 percent registered nurses, but subsequent experience suggested that implementation of the idea required more. One of the most vocal proponents and demonstrators of the effectiveness of the primary nursing-care system is Chief of Nursing Joyce Clifford of Boston's Beth Israel Hospital. Establishing the philosophy that "patients have a right to . . . care . . . personalized . . . planned for and evaluated by a professional registered nurse," she and her colleague, Beth Israel Chief Executive Officer Mitchell Rabkin, MD, implemented primary nursing in 1974. The vast majority of primary nurses there hold the baccalaureate or higher nursing degree.[128] Nursing Dean Luther Christman of Chicago's Rush University, citing the relationship between staffing and patient safety, pointed to the importance of personal accountability and initiative. In the traditional bureaucratic mode of nursing practice, he argued, no one is to blame when things go wrong.[129]

Extending the Scope of Nursing Practice Outside the Hospital

While the various parties argued about how best to nurse patients in hospitals a second debate opened about how to respond to demands for general medical or ambulatory care outside the hospital. The labels attached to this broad public demand for changes in access to health care ranged from "comprehensive" care in the 1950s and 1960s to "primary" care later in the 1960s and 1970s.

The term "primary" health care [not to be confused with primary nursing in hospitals] is an encompassing definition of the provider–patient relationship; it includes the first contact of the patient with a health-care professional, responsibility for longitudinal care, referral and coordinating all aspects of care, health maintenance such as immunizations, and responsibility for teaching about health. Reformers urging the development of a "primary health care system" insisted that access to general health care was lacking and that American citizens had a right to "affordable, accessible" health care.

Widespread political and professional support for the primary health-care movement meant a significant number of people agreed that the hospital-based system left serious gaps to be filled. The public perception in the 1960s was that the existing health-care system was too specialized, too centralized, too impersonal and made care too difficult to obtain.

What was historically unique about the public response to the issue of limited access to health-care services outside the hospital was the emerging consensus that nursing, the largest single health-care group, should expand its scope of practice to provide direct services to patients, including services previously considered solely in the physician's domain. A firm and clear expression of this new view of nursing was made in a 1971 Report to Elliot Richardson, then Secretary of Health, Education and Welfare.

Extending the Scope of Nursing Practice called for nurses in primary care, acute care and long-term care to expand their responsibility to collect medical data and make clinical decisions about patients; it also urged curricular innovations and financial support to modify the education of nurses and physicians toward more collaborative practice. The Secretary's Committee argued that extending the scope of nursing practice was essential to national achievement of the goal of equal access to health services for all citizens. At the same time they acknowledged the tensions between physicians and nurses – ". . . complex and often delicate questions of professional attitudes [are] involved in any consideration of nurses functioning in extended roles."[130]

More surprising, given the strained history between organized medicine and nursing, was the 1970 recommendation of the American Medical Association (AMA) Committee on Nursing, which was subsequently adopted by the AMA. Among other objectives intended to "[increase] the significance of nursing as a primary component in the delivery of medical services," the AMA supported the idea "of expanding the role of the nurse in providing patient care."[131] Edmund Pellegrino, MD, a noted medical education reformer and philosopher, chaired the AMA Committee and was a member of the 1971 Secretary's Committee as well.

These proposals to expand nursing's role were grounded in nursing-care demonstrations carried out in the late 1960s. In the first of these at the University of Colorado, nurse Loretta Ford and physician Henry Silver launched a program "to prepare nurses with bachelor's or master's degrees to assume an expanded role in providing total health care for children."[132] Nurses were expected to provide comprehensive care to well children and identify, appraise, and temporarily manage certain acute and chronic conditions of the sick child. The program intended to prepare nurses for practice in private physicians' offices, clinics and other areas without adequate health services for children.

According to an account of the concept in the *Journal of the American Medical Association*, the nurse was expected to become a colleague of the physician but the basic doctor–nurse relationship and the independence of the physician were to be maintained. The sense of this "expansion" of the nurses' scope of practice one gains from medical accounts is that broadening the nurse's scope was acceptable to progressive-minded physicians as long as the physician retained control in the relationship.

Nurses, of course, objected to these captain-of-the-ship restrictions. Most nurses saw these observational and educational activities as well within the scope of nursing practice and consistent with their long-time public health nursing role.[133]

Public and private experiments mobilizing nurses to assist with perceived shortfalls in health-care delivery continued at a rapid pace in spite of misgivings on the part of physicians who saw threats to their hegemony and nurses who feared "medicalization" of nursing. The federal government funded a series of projects to implement the recommendations of the Secretary's Committee to Study Extended Roles for Nurses. Included among these were the Primex program and other USPHS nursing programs to prepare nurses for primary-care practice. Most of these projects were co-directed by nurses and physicians. However, at that time few were integrated into nursing-school or medical-school curricula; instead they were housed in Continuing Education departments or in Regional Medical Program Offices established under President Lyndon Johnson's Great Society heart, cancer and stroke initiatives. Importantly, innovations in family medicine and the invention of the physician assistant paralleled these efforts to move nursing into broader roles in extra-institutional care.

Attempts to Collaborate

In an attempt to improve dialogue and planning between organized medicine and nursing, the National Joint Practice Commission (NJPC) was established in 1972. The Joint Commission was recommended by the National Commission for the Study of Nursing and Nursing Education; it was supported by grants from the American Medical Association, the American Nurses' Association and the W. K. Kellogg Foundation. From the beginning the NJPC struggled with issues in hospital nursing; its earliest task forces explored care of the aged, rural health delivery, and interdisciplinary education for physicians and nurses.

Kellogg Foundation staffers argued that the high turnover rate in hospital nursing indicated the need for change and that the 700,000 practicing nurses in the US were being used inefficiently. From Kellogg's perspective "the basic issue surrounding the need to examine the roles of nurses and physicians concerns the problem of under-utilization of the professional competence of registered nurses in this country . . . Next to physicians, nurses are trained to function at critical levels of skill encompassing a knowledge of life sciences and clinical expertise."[134]

These efforts to redefine the professional practices of nurses and physicians in the decade immediately following the passage of the Medicare/Medicaid legislation was, of course, a result of pressure on the hospital system created by increased patient access to services and the consequent rising costs of health care. Changing educational patterns for nurses, increased specialization on the part of physicians, a changing social context for women associated with the women's movement, and 1960s civil-rights activism all facilitated nurses' striving to broaden their scope of practice.

Nevertheless, physicians jealously guarded their control over the care of non-hospitalized patients while, at the same time, cautiously supporting expansion of the hospital nurse's role. Inside the hospital, especially in intensive care units, nurses' responsibility for patient-care decisions expanded rapidly.

The federal government encouraged expansion of nurses' roles in intensive care through targeted educational programs under the Regional Medical Programs of the late 1960s and through generous funding of special training courses. But while federal support was crucial to developing nurse practitioner roles in primary-care programs the expansion of nurses' work inside the hospital would probably have gone forward anyway. Rhetoric against intensive care nursing, in spite of the medical prerogatives assumed by nurses, seemed far less vociferous than the medical and nursing resistance to the idea of the nurse practitioner.

A vital distinction between the two movements, of course, was the role of the hospital as arbiter of the intensive care nursing innovations. The nurse caring for patients in the intensive care unit was paid for her/his services by the hospital out of an entirely different insurance source than that which paid the physician. Proliferation and expansion of nursing in these roles had no effect at all on physicians' reimbursement for medical services to hospitalized patients.

No similar strong institutional base (or financial protection for physicians) existed to house and nurture the nursing role in the primary health-care movement. Public-health departments, hospital out-patient departments, neighborhood health centers, voluntary home-nursing agencies, nursing homes, free-standing clinics, and private physicians' offices were the scattered, multi-motivated, often poorly funded bases for primary care. Fully "utilizing the critical skills of nurses," as Kellogg and other planners urged, depended on modification of physicians' lock on payment for out-of-hospital patient-care services. Nursing leader Susan Gortner chided physicians for their insistence on retaining a supervisory role in ambulatory care, asking, "why [is there] an apparent increased need for medical oversight and presence with decreased acuity of illness?"[135]

Still, the primary health-care movement spread during the 1970s era of experimentation in delivering health care. Although continuously controversial, expanding nurses' scope of practice and thus their need for more education became the norm for the seventies. In 1973, arguing that nurses' movement into areas of care traditionally requiring physicians was a growing trend, the Division of Nursing of the USPHS funded a major study of the nurse practitioner movement. The Division of Nursing had invested heavily in education for nurse practitioners; their Longitudinal Study of Nurse Practitioners examined educational programs, students in the programs, and their subsequent employment in "expanded roles."[136] The study reported favorably on the nurse practitioner movement and became a basis for continued funding of training programs for the next ten years.

Mainstream Education for Nurses after 1965

As we saw in the 1950s, the crisis and confusion caused by escalating demands on a small, unprepared workforce set off a series of stop-gap, high-cost efforts to ensure the supply of nurses after hospital expansion began. Plans to train practical nurses, nurse's aides, and to re-train inactive nurses were implemented; at the same time hospitals began to hire far more graduates of their training schools to stay on and work after completing training. The traditional practice of retaining hospital-school graduates to staff the hospitals tended, for a time, to make hospital leaders reluctant to consider giving up their schools. Many hospitals admitted students according to their anticipated staffing needs; their school enrollment grew or shrank depending on their own institutional requirements. But, as noted earlier, hospital schools became increasingly expensive to operate. As external accrediting standards began to be applied and as insurers questioned costs, hospital administrators reconsidered the value of the hospital-owned nursing school.

Meanwhile, educational reformers and planners reconstructing the nation's higher-education system sought ways to enhance and expand the research capability of American universities, admit larger numbers of the middle class to higher education, and upgrade the education of the post-war workforce.[137] Four-year colleges and universities grew steadily but, in a social strategy very significant for nursing, much emphasis was placed on easy, local access to education at the junior or community-college level. The growth of the community college in the 1950s and the problem of educating enough nurses for an expanding hospital system became linked.[138]

Soon nurses were being prepared for "professional nursing practice" in three separate and different educational systems: the hospital-owned, traditional school, which gave a diploma at the end of three years' training; the four-year college program, which was usually a combination of two years of liberal arts and sciences and two or three years of clinical training; and, after 1952, the two-year community-college program which offered a year of arts and sciences and a year of hospital training leading to an associate degree in nursing. All programs required a high school diploma; other admissions standards varied, of course, depending on the quality of the school, the region, and the faculty of the nursing program.

Confronted with this rather peculiar situation nurses and those concerned with nursing struggled to find consensus about the issue that came to be called entry into practice. What was at stake was how well educated the nurse should be to be registered by the state to accept final nursing responsibility for all nursing needed by patients. Hospitals accepted the idea that a professional nurse with a valid state license should be the one responsible. But the question still remained; who was the professional nurse? For sixty years the baccalaureate degree had been proposed but not implemented as the entry standard for state licensure for professional nursing. Virtually all studies about nursing and hospitals were influenced by this enduring and unresolved impasse about the educational standard for entry into professional nursing practice.

In 1965, the American Nurses' Association (ANA) issued a statement on educational preparation for nursing; its so-called Position Paper framed the debate from then on. The ANA Position Paper stipulated three levels of nursing practice: professional, with minimum preparation at the baccalaureate; technical, with minimum preparation at the associate degree; and assistive, prepared in short, pre-service courses in vocational schools. The ANA called for education which would "provide an environment in which the nursing student can develop self-discipline, intellectual curiosity, the ability to think clearly, and acquire the knowledge necessary for practice." The Position Paper insisted that all "education for those who are licensed to practice nursing should take place in institutions of higher education."[139]

Notwithstanding this clear position on the part of nursing's professional organization, movement toward even the last goal was extremely slow. Change was problematic on two levels: it required voluntary closure of local hospital training schools, and, in effect, disenfranchised the licensed practical nurse, who usually had one year of hospital or high-school-based training.

The National Commission for the Study of Nursing and Nursing Education was set up in 1967 to study problems in nursing practice and education. The impetus for the Commission was the set of concerns expressed in the 1963 Secretary's Report *Toward Quality in Nursing*. Paid for by the W. K. Kellogg Foundation, the Avalon Foundation, and a private donor, the Commission was established as a not-for-profit corporation to ensure its freedom from pressure from interest groups. The furor set off by the ANA 1965 Position Paper and the rapid changes in nursing and medical practice during the 1960s guaranteed controversy for the Commission.

The Commission's Report listed a series of familiar points about nursing practice in hospitals and then laid out a set of recommendations: investing in research on nursing practice and advanced training for nurses in physical and biological sciences; a national joint practice commission between medicine and nursing [mentioned earlier]; hospital nursing chiefs to be on par with other administrators and physicians since quality nursing depends on equity among hospital leaders; the baccalaureate as the entry standard for professional practice, and, in its least understood suggestion, the Commission recommended two "related but differing career patterns – episodic and distributive."[140]

The Commission drew heavily on the work of Odin Anderson and sociologist Fred Davis. Quoting Anderson, it argued, "if medical specialists become the model [for nursing practice] the behavioral aspects of patient care will languish and be preempted by lesser trained nurse types . . . if the patient-as-person orientation can be the model, then . . . professional nursing has a viable role model to develop in its educational program."[141] The Commission refuted the supply-side, shortage-inspired solutions of the post-war years, saying that nurses were disenchanted with hospital nursing and that simply producing more nurses solved nothing.

The Lysaught Report, as it came to be called (after its director, Jerome Lysaught of the University of Rochester in New York State), attracted much attention in 1970. The Commission continued to issue pamphlets and report at conferences for a year or two. The W. K. Kellogg Foundation relied on the Commission's findings as a guide for part of its funding for nursing projects in the 1970s.

But some nurse leaders, both in hospital nursing and in education, stood to lose status if the baccalaureate standard was adopted. In many cases, leaders in hospital nursing identified first with the hospitals where they had responsibility. Changing the educational standard for entry, they feared, would make recruitment of nurses more difficult, make the hospital's school obsolete, and ultimately raise personnel costs. Nurse educators in hospital schools and community colleges and their alumnae also had much to lose: their schools, their prestige, and their identity as professional nurses.

In addition to the fears of hospital and nurse leaders and alumnae, saving the traditional hospital schools was very important to hospital board members, physicians loyal to the hospital schools, and community leaders who saw professionalizing, university-based "outsiders" threatening the freedom and autonomy of their community hospitals.

Earlier pre- and post-World War II decisions to use the accrediting mechanisms in nursing to "lift all boats" – i.e. preserve as many schools as possible – tended to keep many small schools in the system. This may have prevented the better, stronger schools from attracting resources and growing toward efficiency.

In a 1985 interview, Esther Lucile Brown, who had been one of the architects of the 1950s nursing agenda, reconsidered the "lift all boats" approach of post-war accreditation programs. In hindsight, she thought, it might have been better to "leave the situation alone" and allow only the better institutions to survive. In other words, nursing schools should have been faced with a "sink or swim" ultimatum. It is hard to imagine how the weak post-war nursing organizations could have implemented such a draconian approach in the face of strong hospital and medical pressure to produce more nurses.[142]

The nursing-education decision of mid-century, i.e. to preserve as many schools as possible, was exactly opposite to that of Flexner-era medicine fifty years earlier, which closed many marginal, non-conforming medical schools and reduced the supply of physicians.[143] Turn-of-the-century medical academicians sought science-based education and better students while practitioners also began to embrace science and reduce overcrowding in the profession. Their emerging consensus got a great impetus from the Carnegie Foundation-supported Flexner Report of 1910, which was devastatingly critical of non-university-based medical schools. Its popularity led weaker medical schools to close at a fast rate and philanthropists to fund university-based medical schools.

It would be 1982, almost twenty years after the ANA's 1965 resolution, before the National League for Nursing, the accrediting body for nurse education programs including those run by hospitals, could fully commit itself to the baccalaureate standard for entry into professional nursing. Brown, reflecting on her forty-year involvement with American nursing, rather ruefully noted that nursing leaders took a whole generation to act in an unequivocal way on the issue of the baccalaureate as the qualification for nursing.[144] She recalled that "they couldn't find it in their hearts" to create the rancor change would cause among them, and feared stratifying nursing.[145]

Of course, as we have seen, nursing was already stratified by the variously prepared caregivers called in to staff the nation's hospitals. Team nursing and other task-oriented patient-care strategies struggled to deal with the care problem created by undifferentiated patient-care responsibilities of baccalaureate graduates, nurses graduating from the other two types of programs, and additional personnel trained in various ways to assist professional nurses. The crucial basis of the quality problem in nursing, of course, was the education system's inability to produce enough fully prepared nurses. Moreover, the hospitals' labor policies meant they were not retaining nurses long enough to gain experience and satisfy the hospitals' own demands for highly skilled nurses.

Third-party payers for hospital services, who grew more and more important in every health-care decision after 1950, probably did as much as anyone to help dismantle the hospital nursing-school system by their reluctance to allow hospitals to pass through the costs of the schools as patient-care expenses. By the 1960s even very prosperous hospitals found that owning and operating these schools was a financial burden. But setting the entry standard for professional nursing at the baccalaureate level also worried insurers. The costs of nursing, always factored into the charge for the hospital patient room, were invariably cited as the main reason for higher demands for reimbursement from third parties by hospitals. Although costs for renovation and installing new technology were absorbed as necessary business expenses, raising the standard of education for professional practice and therefore the salaries of professional nurses, insurers feared, would drive daily room charges up. To those using this logic, the low "cost per trained nurse" of Associate Degree nurses was attractive since they assumed these nurses would demand less money than more highly-educated nurses.

Public Support for Nursing Education

The Associate Degree in Nursing offered by community colleges put the costs of nursing education squarely on the shoulders of tax-payers and the students. By the 1970s hospitals and the insurance industry experienced considerable relief from the costs of educating entry-level nurses.

The federal government, through the United States Public Health Service (USPHS), and other agencies such as the National Institute of Mental Health, invested huge sums in nursing education, beginning in 1946 but most generously after 1964. By 1970 nursing schools grew to accommodate 5,000 additional students; $15.4 million had been given to schools to improve training; 30,000 nurses received tuition support under the Professional Nurse Traineeship Program; $73 million in construction grants was spent and $103 million was dedicated to training nurse administrators and supervisors.[146]

Eventually these federal investments in nursing attracted critics. Economist Uwe Reinhardt, for instance, questioned the logic of subsidizing education for health professionals and, at the same time, attempting to control costs in the health-care system. Whether or not his position was feasible in the face of incessant demand for nurses, Reinhardt still asked the right question: "are we willing to pay for the manpower we are now supplying and will be supplying in the future?"[147] Similar expansionist proposals in medical education were also being questioned and cautioned against as costs for health care began to mount.[148]

The leaders in the Division of Nursing at the USPHS who were orchestrating the post-war reform of the nursing-education system wanted to focus their investment on higher education for nurses. They were often forced, however, to extend their grants and loans to hospital-based training schools because of political pressure from hospital constituencies. One example was the capitation-grant program for schools of nursing authorized under the Nurse Training Act of 1971, which distributed money during the 1970s on the basis of growth in the number of students enrolled in schools. These funds were distributed to all schools accredited by the National League for Nursing. Thus hospital-based schools were eligible; the formulas for fund distribution favored the baccalaureate and associate degree programs.[149] National and state hospital associations continued to insist that the federal government treat all suppliers of nurses alike.

Ultimately the hospital schools declined in importance. The remarkable expansion of nursing in America's community colleges in the 1960s and 1970s, on the other hand, is testimony not only to the demand for nurses but also to the enthusiasm of community-college presidents for nursing programs. Nursing programs added prestige to community colleges because they were higher in level than other vocational programs. Like hospital schools, they became locally popular providers of a vital resource as they consistently attracted students who were immediately employable upon graduation. Also attracted to the two-year nurse-education programs were private philanthropy and health-system planners who saw in the community-college movement a way to staff the hospitals, retain traditional local commitment to nursing education, and contain the costs of the hospital system.[150] The idea of a stepped approach to higher levels of nursing, i.e. two years to qualify for entry to practice, followed by supplementary education for advancement, appealed to some planners as a way to obtain large numbers of low-cost, entry-level nurses. This "ladder" approach relied on attrition or failure of nurses to seek more education to ensure that not too many nurses would be seeking higher-paying positions. The "ladder" would later be characterized as a "trickle up" approach to creating an appropriate mix of nurses.

Nursing and Social Mobility

Allied with, and implicit in, easy applicant access to nursing is the persistent idea that one of nursing's social functions is to be a vehicle for social mobility for women [and sometimes men] with fewer employment opportunities. Over time those said to be seeking a better life through nursing have been variously identified as women from rural areas, working-class families, minorities, or older people needing new careers.

Eli Ginzberg is a frequent exponent of nursing's social-mobility function.[151] In the late 1970s Ginzberg's position sounded especially strong. Having made the point that hospital administrators were hiring more better-trained and experienced nurses and fewer associate-degree (two-year) nurses, Ginzberg argued that such a move on the part of hospitals could lead to "major [social] conflict; . . . it is essential that, at a minimum, these calculations of opportunity and equity be factored into all decision-making . . . [which might] alter the existing and prospective educational and employment structures for nursing."[152] The link between nursing and attaining social equity was made often during the 1970s. Much of the rhetoric seemed to assume that minority or other disadvantaged persons' entry into nursing could only be at the bottom rung of the "stepped approach" or educational ladder. This "bottom rung" perspective was not an issue when it came to minority access to medicine, law, or other single-entry occupations.[153] As time went on, however, minorities, especially Asians and African Americans, who entered professional nursing programs chose baccalaureate education more often than other basic programs.[154]

Adapting Nursing Education to the Times

By the 1970s the associate-degree movement was booming; its leaders were not eager to see it become the focal point for nursing's social-equity assignment. Citing calls for opening more and different opportunities in nursing, some nurses took care to point out nursing's historic vulnerability, i.e. being asked to spearhead otherwise unattainable social goals. While embracing the idea of an open curriculum and greater flexibility in entering and completing education for nursing they argued for careful study to select realistic curricula and check the actual outcomes of educational innovations.[155]

Experiments with ungraded courses, programmed or self instruction, open enrollment and generally less rigorous standards characterized new thinking in education at the turn of the seventies. Students graduating from undemanding nursing programs were, however, still held to the requirement that they should be able to pass licensure examinations, immediately perform as professional nurses, and meet hospital practice standards. Many could not do it. This was a problem for graduates of both four- and two-year experimental nursing programs. At the time, it hit two-year programs harder because they attracted a heterogeneous student body in terms of academic skills and the students had to learn a great deal in a very brief time. Nursing-student failures on the so-called state boards, the standard exams for state licensure, began to be an issue.[156]

Baccalaureate programs had problems too. Implementation of the baccalaureate entry standard for professional nursing was inhibited by the need to convince recruits to nursing and their families that investing in four years of college education would show a reasonable return. Low wages and trying working conditions for much of the period between 1950 and 1970 made nursing a less than attractive option for the college-bound student. However, in the early seventies nursing salaries finally began to rise and drew abreast of entry earnings of graduates in the social sciences and humanities.[157]

The nagging myth that nurses normally worked for only a few years before marriage also hampered interest in investing in college degrees. Notwithstanding this common misconception, nursing career years after graduation increased steadily throughout the years after World War II. In 1972 88 percent of divorced or separated and single nurses were employed in nursing; 69 percent of widows and 66 percent of married nurses were active. Although the age group 30–34 worked less than any other, 60 percent of them were practicing.[158]

The women's movement of the 1960s and 1970s did not readily embrace nursing; in fact, the nursing profession was sharply criticized by some feminists, who thought nursing promulgated negative female stereotypes. Nevertheless, the environment created by the broader women's movement did help improve access to higher education for a wider spectrum of women, including nurses. As salaries crept up and then began to be attractive it became easier to show the career feasibility of the baccalaureate degree to women and men interested in nursing careers.

Essential Links between Education and Practice

But the lag in creating baccalaureate programs that produced truly effective clinical nurses with advanced knowledge and skills delayed the identification of the baccalaureate graduate as the best clinical nurse, one who should actually be the standard. During the immediate post-war period baccalaureate programs turned out teachers and administrators for schools and hospitals. These programs, which usually recruited holders of hospital nursing diplomas, did not emphasize unique clinical training for their students. Their goal was to fill the ranks of faculty and nursing-service administrators. Their generic graduates, that is those who enrolled with no previous nursing preparation, were not impressively better practitioners than diploma or even associate-degree graduates. It was late in the 1960s before clinical courses of sufficient quality to meet hospital nursing demands became common in baccalaureate programs. It is possible that the associate-degree movement, with its innovations and resources, siphoned off many of the scarce nurse-educators who would have more quickly developed better clinical content for baccalaureate programs.

Here again, we should recall the reciprocal relationship between practice and education in a practice-based discipline such as nursing. Changing nursing practices and the new knowledge requirements they created fueled improvements in baccalaureate programs by demonstrating just what their graduates needed to know. In the 1970s, nursing specialties, in psychiatry, oncology, critical care, nurse practitioner practices, midwifery and others, became codified in programs offering master's degrees which increasingly became accepted as the credential for specialty practice in nursing. This new understanding of the work at the advanced level of nursing practice helped define the generalist baccalaureate nurse more clearly and gave coherence to the curricula by clarifying which basic courses were essential and what clinical knowledge was common to the broad spectrum of nursing practice.[159]

The so-called "unification" movement between nursing education and practice on medical-center campuses was fueled by the deep concern felt by many nurses about the separation of nursing education from its practice base. One high cost of transferring education for nurses away from hospital schools was geographic, psychological and experiential distance between teachers, students and clinicians. In 1956, Dorothy Smith, an innovative and far-sighted dean, unified her university school of nursing with the hospital nursing-care system at the University of Florida in Gainesville. Although the Florida experiment failed after a few years, Smith's demonstration paved the way for changes in university-based education which followed more than a decade later. Case Western Reserve University's Frances Payne Bolton School of Nursing, aided by federal funding, launched its "Experiment in Nursing" in 1969. The University of Rochester (New York), and Rush University in Chicago created their own versions of the concept in 1972. The central idea was to encourage academic nurse faculty to accept responsibility for patient care while sustaining their academic teaching and research work, thus bringing the benefits of their scholarship to bear on patient care. Clinically based and focused teaching and "faculty practice" thus became, during the late seventies and eighties, a restored nursing ideal.

In 1981 the Robert Wood Johnson Foundation in Princeton, New Jersey, funded an eight-year project to try to link, in a similar way, schools of nursing with nursing homes. Although successful in its implementation, this version of the "unification" idea continues to be hampered by limited financial support for long-term care.[160] Nursing homes, unlike hospitals, do not have the resources to invest in or share the cost of education. For, in addition to its care and education advantages, unifying nursing education and practice also offered nursing schools the chance to underwrite some of the costs of education. Faculty salaries could be partially funded by patient-care revenues even though faculty usually remained employees of the university. Furthermore, faculty access to clinical patient services in hospitals and other settings facilitated their opportunity to do clinically-focused research.

Nursing education, after the passage of the 1965 Medicare and Medicaid legislation, continued to be torn by conflicting goals. New patient-care needs coupled with higher standards for traditional nursing care and combined with academic ambition required better-educated nurses; faith in tradition, vested interests, social-equity concerns and fear of nursing shortage pulled the opposite way toward continuing the status quo with its supply-side educational strategies. Through it all new nurses kept pouring out of the system; the number of registered nurses per 100,000 population doubled between 1960 and 1980 (see table 3.1).

Emerging Specialism

Some nurses chose to limit their practice to specialty areas almost from the beginning of organized nursing. Public health nurses, nurse anesthetists, and nurse midwives defined themselves and practiced as specialists throughout the twentieth century. And, as nurse historian Bonnie Bullough points out, before World War II nurses sought "post-graduate" training in a variety of specialty areas from obstetrics to nursing management.[161] These nurses, who had sometimes graduated from mediocre hospital training programs, sought short courses offered by larger hospitals to make up for lacks in their own programs, to improve their competitiveness as private duty nurses, or to become nursing supervisors.

But specialization in nursing really boomed in the rapidly changing health-care environment of the 1960s. First of all, the money was there to support differentiation of practice. Historian George Rosen clarified the connection between specialization and affluence in 1944. As he phrased it, "differentiation among healers is dependent on economic conditions . . . the accumulation of an economic surplus [enables] the society to support them while they are carrying on their professional activities."[162] Of course, Rosen was speaking of the specialism that swept medicine in the 1930s and 1940s. Twenty-five years later Lyndon Johnson's Great Society programs and American affluence afforded nursing an economic base to support its own differentiation. Changing patterns of work, new technology, higher public expectations of the health-care system, and professional ambitions spurred nurses to select specific arenas of nursing practice in which to develop their individual careers.

The emergence of psychiatric nursing after World War II, for example, was encouraged by public concern about widespread mental illness revealed among those serving in the military. The National Mental Health Act of 1946 helped support nurses who chose to obtain graduate degrees focused on psychiatric mental-health nursing. Nurses took advantage of the public funds available for higher education, and nurse specialists in psychiatric mental-health nursing soon appeared and began to develop a wide array of specialized practices.

The intensive care movement created specialties in both medicine and nursing. The impact was proportionately greater in nursing since such large numbers of intensive care nurses were needed to staff units in virtually every American hospital.[163] Now called critical-care nursing, the specialty has been led by the American Association of Critical-Care Nurses (AACN) since 1969; it is the largest of all nursing specialty groups at more than 80,000 members. Similarly, nurses specializing in the care of cancer patients banded together in 1975 to form the Oncology Nursing Society (ONS). Like the AACN, the cancer nurses organized to set and promote standards of practice, to support study and research in their specialty and to educate for practice in their field. Other groups, such as the nephrology nurses and the emergency room nurses, did the same.

Eventually, these nurse specialists came to fit into the categories "intensivists" and "consulting nurse specialists" coined by Aiken in her 1990 analysis of hospital nursing.[164] The developmental process was a complicated one which took slightly different forms among the various areas of practice. Initially, most nurses who specialized learned their skills on the job. The evolution of critical-care nurses, nephrology nurses and oncology nurses sounds very similar when recalled by nurses who pioneered the fields. At first a few nurses collaborated with physicians in the specialty to decide who would do what in patient care; nurses in the various specialties later met one another at medical meetings where they went to learn more about clinical innovations. Critical-care nurses, oncology nurses and nephrology nurses all trace their own specialty organizations to nurse groups that evolved as a result of interested nurses collecting together at medical meetings.

The first nurses trained their successors via the apprentice method and later through educational programs based in hospital and medical specialty organizations. Some of these programs were underwritten by federal or private foundation funds; some were very informal demonstrations, e.g. over the patient's bed. In the beginning the recognized competence of an individual nurse specialist was based on accomplishment since there were no credentialing mechanisms.

After the specialty organizations developed, many began to set standards and develop certification systems for their respective specialties as did the American College of Nurse-Midwives in 1971, the critical-care nurses (AACN) in 1976, and the National Board of Pediatric Nurse Practitioners and Associates in 1977. The pioneer certifying group in nursing was the American Association of Nurse Anesthetists (AANA); they began certifying in 1946. The question in credentialing is: who will authorize and guarantee competent practice within the specialty framework? Will it be the larger professional organization, i.e. the American Nurses' Association, the specialty organization, or the state? The issue is open and, at the moment, all three avenues are employed to varying degrees by nurses seeking specialty credentials. Increasingly, as we have seen, the master's degree in nursing is the essential credential to sit for specific certifying exams.

In 1976, educator Shirley Smoyak traced the first ten years of post-war nursing specialty growth in *Nursing Outlook*.[165] As early as 1952 the National League for Nursing decided to place specialty preparation at the master's level. As Smoyak points out, however, for some fifteen years master's programs in nursing actually contained very little clinical content, focusing instead on teacher training and administration. It wasn't until after 1963, when *Toward Quality in Nursing* set in motion the chain of political decisions dedicating federal dollars to train clinical nursing specialists, that clinical training at the master's level began to spread.

One function of clinical specialization was to keep experienced, talented nurses at the bedside working in direct patient care. The idea of advanced practice caught on after some initial delay during which these expert nurses figured out what their jobs were. Even after the federal money began to dry up in the Nixon years, graduations from specialty master's programs continued to grow. One estimate suggests that, in the three years between 1977 and 1980, the number of clinical nurse specialists jumped from 9,928 to 17,626 and the number of nurse practitioners and midwives grew from 3,296 to 5,500.[166]

The nurse–specialist phenomenon is reminiscent of the history of specialization in medicine. Many nurses were skeptical of early nurse specialists, thinking they were becoming too medical and abandoning the broad, caring role of nursing. This is similar to early twentieth-century criticism leveled at medical specialists for abandoning their obligation to know and practice general medicine.[167] It certainly does seem that the specialism of medicine influenced the specialism of nursing. Clinical nurse specialists and nurse practitioners sought to fill the gaps in care left when physicians specialized; alternatively, they took up new work created when new care modalities appeared.

Nephrology nursing, for instance, grew out of new treatments for kidney failure, renal dialysis, and the later renal transplantations. These treatments created a whole new class of patients with complex needs for nursing care. On the other hand, as we have seen, nurse practitioners gained support based on their ability to provide general care to a public which felt deprived of primary care services, which seemed less available as medicine specialized.[168]

More established specialties such as nurse midwives and nurse anesthetists sorted out their practice opportunities in protracted struggles with physicians. Both of these latter groups grew stronger during the period because they could offer good clinical care acceptable to patients at a reasonable fee.

Nursing specialization was characterized by an experimental attitude. Especially in the formative years (1970s) new nurse specialists and nurse practitioners tended to experiment with new roles and adapt both their practice and education for practice based on their experiences. Rather than following any grand design they tested ideas and responses and, in general, moved into areas of least resistance. Late in this period gerontologic nurse practitioners and specialists began to appear in response to the prevailing sense of crisis around care of the elderly.[169]

Expansion and Differentiation

After the Medicare and Medicaid legislation of 1965 a major effort to redefine and expand nursing's scope of practice spread across the spectrum of patient care from intensive care in hospitals to ambulatory care and to patients' homes. Variously called clinical specialists, nurse practitioners, and nurse clinicians, those who worked in these roles redefined the nurse–physician working relationship. The physician became more sharply defined as the

diagnostic, therapeutic specialist while the nurse focused on observation, intervention, coordination of care, and teaching patients.
Conflict over control of practice, and debate over whether the nurse
substituted for the physician or complemented his/her work, characterized the period.[170]

By the 1970s the impact of a decade of federal subsidies for higher
education for nurses began to be felt as better-prepared faculty and
clinicians entered the nursing market. Rapprochement between
nursing educators and nurses in practice was accelerated by the
unification movement and the introduction of clinical specialists in
hospital practice. The most growth occurred at the associate-degree
level although baccalaureate, master's, and doctoral programs began
expanding rapidly.[171] The impasse over establishing a single entry
point to professional nursing practice continued in spite of constant
efforts to come to a resolution.[172]

Most nurses continued to practice in hospitals – the proportion
averaged between 65 and 70 percent. More and more hospital
nurses specialized and assumed more clinical responsibility. Nurses
did migrate to home care and specialty practice but did not move to
nursing homes in large numbers in spite of efforts to revise the
curriculum and demonstrate the rewards of nursing practice with
the frail elderly. Resources to pay nurses in nursing homes did not
materialize in spite of exponential growth in nursing-home beds
over the period after 1965.

During the 20 years between 1963 and 1982 the number of
nursing homes nearly doubled. A substantial segment of nursing-
home expansion occurred in the for-profit, private sector. An aging
population, falling length of stay in acute-care hospitals, and available money for institutional care locked in the acute-care sector
yielded a vicious combination of higher demand for long-term care
and marginal, financially strapped institutions.[173] In 1990 about half
the care in nursing homes was purchased privately; the other
half was paid by Medicaid or other third-party sources.

The expanded scope of nursing practice and redefinition of the
nurse–physician working relationship has combined with a radically
enlarged nursing workforce to change the face of hospital nursing
in the years after 1965. But major problems continued in the distribution of nurses across the care system, that is, in hospitals, home
care and long-term care, while deep disagreements about initial
preparation for professional practice have dogged both the profession and those concerned about caregivers for the nation.

3

Relocating Care, 1980–1995

No Simple Answers

The forty-year period under discussion here frames the central-ization of nursing care in hospitals and efforts to relocate patient care and thus nursing to other settings. In the 1990s health-care plan-ners are poised to send more of the sick, injured and dependent back to their own homes or arrange care for them in other, less costly care systems. This de-emphasis of institutions has already affected other sectors of health care, most notably public hospitals and institutions for the care of the mentally ill. Intense focus on retrenchment in the size and function of community acute-care hospitals, that is, a significant debate about relocating care of the acutely ill, insured patient did not begin until the late 1980s and early 1990s.

Instead, during most of the 1980s effort was directed to reducing patients' length of stay in hospitals and managing in-patient care within the framework of prospective reimbursement under the DRG (diagnostically related group) method of payment. These tactics tended to create higher levels of acuity among the patients who remained in hospitals, with the unanticipated consequence of requiring more nursing; this outcome surprised and, at first, seemed to baffle hospital managers.

The 1983 Institute of Medicine (IOM) study, *Nursing and Nursing Education: Public Policies and Private Actions,* was originally mandated by the federal Nurse Training Act Amendments of 1979 and finally commissioned in 1981.[174] The IOM study grew out of earlier criticisms leveled by economist Uwe Reinhardt and others at large federal expenditures on nursing education ($1.6 billion since 1964). Several successive administrations had tried to curtail spending but nursing's Congressional supporters prevailed. Substantial levels of funding for nursing education survived in spite of cutbacks by both the Nixon and Carter administrations. The effect of the cutbacks was to reduce direct support of students; however, expansion of programs to prepare more nurses, especially those graduating nurse practitioners, nurse-midwives, and other specialists, was encouraged.

The charge to the 1983 IOM committee was to investigate three questions: whether there was continued need for federal support, how to get nurses into "medically underserved areas," and, last, how to "encourage nurses to remain active in their profession."[175] This last charge to the IOM panel was grounded in the enduring myth that nurses work a few years in their profession and then drop out or switch fields. This, in spite of the fact that, at the time of the study, 76 percent of all nurses were actively practicing.

The IOM found that nurses who weren't working (about 24 percent) usually dropped out for personal or family reasons, not because they took non-nursing jobs. By the early 1980s turnover rates in hospital nursing had fallen to around 30 percent from the high levels (67 percent at one point) of the 1950s and 1960s. The IOM found that nurses' dissatisfaction with working conditions focused on matters related to scope of practice and role definition as well as job strain and mental and physical fatigue.

In its recommendations relative to funding education, the IOM re-visited and, indeed, seemed to insist on preserving the "social mobility" function of nursing noted in the policies of earlier decades. Hoping to maintain a steady supply of new graduates in nursing, while at the same time improving the quality of the nurse work-force, the IOM panel refused to recommend a single educational standard for entry to the occupation. Instead, they called for maintaining easy access to nursing jobs and continuous subsequent re-training of graduate nurses.

The language of their recommendation is reluctant, even rueful; "Although not an approach preferred . . . in terms of time and cost, attainment of future supply goals may well depend on a continual upgrading of the quality of a pool of nurses that is primarily nourished by streams of new entrants whose initial career objective may have been merely to secure nursing employment at minimum personal cost."[176]

At the same time, however, the IOM panel called for increased support of nursing education in master's programs, including more funds for preparing nurse practitioners. They also urged federal and state support for nurses at all levels who would work in long-term care, especially nursing homes. But, noting that "[the] labor market cannot function properly when there are financial, geographic and other barriers to the provision of medical care and health services," the panel cautioned that increasing numbers of nurses would not, by itself, alter the problem of medically underserved areas. The causes of maldistribution of nurses as well as other medical services, they argued, rested in the nation's health-care financing arrangements.[177]

The IOM study was one of the most sophisticated and well documented studies of nursing of the last fifty years. Clearly documented information on nursing and detailed justification of each recommendation contrasts with the "expert opinion" character and limited detail of many earlier studies. Nevertheless, the IOM panel was embarrassingly wrong about the future supply of generalist nurses, predicting that the "aggregate supply and demand for generalist nurses [will] be in reasonable balance during this decade [referring to the 1980s]."[178] Financial support for entry-level nurse education to prime the pump of nurse supply seemed to them to be unnecessary.

To be fair, the IOM collected and reviewed its data during the 1982–83 recession and in a pre-DRG nursing environment. Few fully appreciated the critical shortage of nurses that would develop after prospective reimbursement (DRGs) "speeded up" the movement of patients through America's hospitals. Intensification of hospital patients' nursing needs created a nursing shortage by requiring still higher ratios of nurses to patients. And these nurses had to be fully prepared to quickly meet each patient's care needs. Hospital managers soon believed they faced a crisis, and sought relief.

And so, five years later, the Secretary's Commission on Nursing was appointed to ascertain whether there was a true shortage of nurses in hospitals. They reported in 1988 that, indeed, shortage was once more an issue.[179] A study of hospitals which were successful in attracting nurses, the so-called "magnet hospitals," helped set the stage for the Secretary's Commission Final Report.[180] Saying that the nursing shortage was "real, widespread, and of significant magnitude," the Commission attributed part of the problem to poor utilization of professional nurses by hospitals. The Commission argued that the shortage was caused, not by too few nurses, but by constantly rising demand for more nurses on the part of hospitals.

And further, they pointed out that nurses were a bargain for hospitals (but not for society), since artificially low pay made nurses all-purpose employees hospitals could and did hire to do everything, thus wasting a needed public resource.

The observation of the Secretary's Commission was in no way novel, but clearly this is one labor lesson that is hard to learn. Twenty-five years earlier, in 1963, economist Donald Yett explained that an increased supply of nurses led to large relative salary declines, which then led to shortages.[181] In 1971 Stuart Altman argued that, if wages were restrained from rising above the level where supply equals demand, ". . . employers will wish to hire more workers at this artificially low wage than are available."[182] Once again, in 1987, Linda Aiken pointed out that the narrow difference between the salaries of professional nurses and those of practical nurses or aides made hospitals prefer to hire professional nurses as all-purpose workers, thus accelerating a perceived shortage.[183]

Predictably, the 1988 Commission forecast a continued rising demand for nurses and made a series of recommendations to address the situation. They called for better utilization of nurses' time through modifying staffing patterns and improved use of assistants and technology. At the same time, they called for higher pay for nurses, especially targeted to relieve chronic wage compression, which, they said, discouraged experienced nurses from continuous hospital practice, since accumulating seniority only marginally improved nurses' income. They urged that nurses be more involved in high-level decision-making in institutions which were delivering nursing care. Finally, departing from the 1983 IOM panel's stance, the Secretary's Commission thought more financial aid should go to undergraduate as well as graduate nursing students. In recommending more investment in entry-level nursing education the Secretary's Commission returned to a policy position out of favor since early in the seventies.

The shortage of hospital nurses in the late 1980s set off another blizzard of commentary and articles in both the professional and the popular press. Familiar and not-so-familiar names appear; Eli Ginzberg, from whom we first heard in 1948, argued that higher salaries for nurses would attract new recruits to nursing, especially minority candidates, and would hold nurses at work or cause them to return. Although by this time it was understood that the labor force participation of nurses was the highest among women's occupations, many commentators continued to suggest that unemployed nurses were "out there someplace" just waiting for higher salaries. Ginzberg and others also hoped that nursing leaders would drop their campaign to make the bachelor's degree the standard for entry, implying that campaigns to raise entry standards contributed to the shortage.[184]

Taking an opposite tack, Linda Aiken cited falling length of stay among hospital patients, rising in-patient severity of illness and complex demands on hospital nurses to show that, more than ever, nurses required better base preparation for hospital practice.[185] Extending and detailing this idea, Karen Zander listed hospital nurses' responsibilities: recognizing and treating patient complications related to treatment, detecting unanticipated complications unrelated to treatment, and handling complications related to self care and extensions of known disease processes. Using new language for the traditional, familiar coordination function of nurses, she described "managed care within acute care." The nurse's job, she argued, blends the efforts of physicians and other caregivers to secure the best interests of the hospitalized patient. Zander explicitly linked these functions to hospital costs and income.[186]

The Zander and Aiken argument was buttressed by earlier investigations of hospital care of critically ill patients. In 1986, the studies by Knaus et al. of the relationship between shared nurse–physician decision-making and patient welfare provided ammunition for nurses' arguments that patient safety and survival depended on fully prepared and sufficient hospital nurses. According to Knaus, the hospital with the best mortality rate was the one that cancelled major elective surgery if the nursing staff was insufficient; the unit nurse in charge made the cancellation decision.[187] The 1980s debate about quality reflected the decades-long struggle to balance demands for plenty of low-cost nurses to staff hospitals with the necessity for high-quality nursing practiced by persons enjoying full mastery of their clinical fields.

In 1987 Claire Fagin accurately forecast the severe nursing shortage then on the horizon. Attributing part of the problem to "the confused educational system," she called attention to the continuing trend toward over-production of associate-degree and licensed vocational nurses and under-production of baccalaureate and higher-degree nurses.[188] The public's willingness to support graduate education for clinical specialists and refusal to support baccalaureate education, she argued, created an impossible or at least an eccentric educational sequence for preparing highly skilled nurses. Access to graduate school required the academic base of the baccalaureate; too many nurses prepared without that base constricted the supply of clinical specialists and nurse practitioners.

In 1988, 35 percent of nursing students enrolled in baccalaureate programs, 55 percent in associate-degree programs and 10 percent still enrolled in hospital-based programs. By 1993 some change in the direction sought by Fagin began to appear; 41 percent of nursing students were enrolled in baccalaureate programs, 51 percent in associate-degree programs, and 8 percent in hospital-based programs. Of 88,149 nursing graduates in 1993, 24,442 held the baccalaureate, an increase of 14 percent over the previous year. In 1994, baccalaureate graduations jumped another 16 percent.[189]

Enrollment in master's degree nursing programs also trended upward especially after the late 1980s. A sharp upward turn of nearly 11 percent in 1994/95 seemed to reflect nurses' recognition of the utility of investing in education to grasp opportunities in advanced practice positions. About 30 percent of the 1994/95 master's enrollees (30,718) pursued study as nurse practitioners while another 3 percent sought training as nurse-midwives or nurse anesthetists.[190]

It is difficult to say whether the baccalaureate trends will be lasting and whether first applicants to nursing schools chose the baccalaureate route on the basis of recognition of a changed career trajectory in the field. Certainly the overall rise in enrollments shows no change in the supply-side nursing-education practices of previous decades. Aiken, in particular, is critical of the educational complexity and waste associated with the "trickle up" approach to preparing highly skilled nurses. She and her colleagues argue that the educational mix now being produced is still much too thin for the care requirements of the present and the future.[191]

Nurses who entered the profession with an associate degree or a hospital diploma in the 1980s did face a daunting series of educational and experiential hurdles limiting, or at least complicating, their access to specialized training and advanced practice positions, i.e. advancement in the field. They found themselves competing with traditional, high-achieving high school graduates for slots in baccalaureate programs and later competing with those same baccalaureate graduates for spaces in master's programs. The improved status and pay of the nursing career created a more competitive environment and easy access to nursing becomes, for some, an illusion rather than an opportunity. Their frustration and disillusion is easy to understand.[192]

For colleges offering higher education for nurses, multiple entry points to the field mean making a continuing investment in special training in sciences and clinical content for nurses prepared in associate-degree and hospital-based programs. Many baccalaureate programs accommodate generic four-year matriculants, students holding associate degrees, students holding diplomas from hospital-based schools, and students with degrees in other fields who seek nursing as a second career. A significant portion of the baccalaureate educational enterprise is used to add needed theory and experience omitted in shorter entry programs so that all baccalaureate graduates will be able to participate in the current job market and qualify for advanced practice training if they desire to do so. In 1994, of the 133,464 students enrolled in bachelor's-degree nursing programs, 36,192 were two-year associate-degree or hospital-diploma registered nurses returning to school for the baccalaureate degree. Many hospitals offer tuition as an employee benefit, making return to school possible. Of course, this practice re-attaches the cost of educating nurses to the cost of patient care.

The Changing Marketplace

The nursing marketplace changed as positions in hospitals became less numerous for entry-level nurses. Rapid job growth is in home care, ambulatory care, and other arenas where a baccalaureate degree or higher may be required as the entry credential. Typically, practice in out-of-hospital settings is quite independent; consultation with senior nurses is by phone or after-the-fact conference. Thus nurses with more education and experience are sought for these now more responsible and demanding positions.[193]

Meanwhile, the reduction in beds and downsizing of hospital staffs through layoffs and attrition generated the establishment of a new federal commission in April 1994. Alarmed that hospitals are trimming their workforce, and seeking to find if the quality of hospital patient care is suffering, the Institute of Medicine (IOM) was authorized by Congress to do still another study. The intent of the study is to determine "to what extent there is a need for an increase in the number of nurses in hospitals and nursing homes in order to promote the quality of patient care and reduce the incidence among nurses of work-related injuries and stress."[194] The IOM is due to report the findings of this study in mid-1996. The work of the study is often characterized as investigating the problems created by implementing the recommendations of the 1988 IOM study which called for reassigning the non-nurse duties often delegated to nurses.[195]

This problem in building a nursing workforce well matched to late twentieth-century care needs is in interesting contrast to the concerns voiced about the physician supply. In medicine, the concern is about preparing too many specialists; critics say the "trickle down" theory has failed. The hope of the 1970s and 1980s that preparing a larger number of physicians would yield better dispersion of physicians and improved access to care has not materialized.

At some risk of over-simplifying, we observe that the United States has, for some time, been under-educating the bulk of our nurses and over-educating too many of our physicians in relation to the nation's health-care needs.[196] The primary-care emphasis and preference for out-of-hospital treatment exhibited by managed care companies exacerbates these health-manpower concerns. Finding a new balance will take considerable time as we sort through the implications of recent approaches to caring for America's citizens. Managed care, reducing overall costs, and shifting the financial risk to providers of care will set in motion a string of unpredictable consequences to care itself and to those who provide it.

Context for Future Issues

Returning to the original proposition that post-World War II growth and development of nursing and hospitals depended on each other, it is clear that hospitals and nurses were influenced by changes in social attitudes about health care, medical and scientific imperatives, and a host of other contextual stimuli including how care of the sick would be paid for. Nursing care was tantamount to hospital care; during the last forty years both worker and workplace were transformed; they adapted and adjusted to sweeping social, political and economic change.

The relationship between nursing and hospitals is a by-product of the peculiar nature of hospitals' recent history. After World War II, hospitals promised a consuming American public a special, centralized place for medical care replete with state-of-the-art technology. In the 1950s political scientist Herman Finer warned that local, community hospitals were in a monopolistic position and could control both the quality and quantity of their services from "consumer contrived" rather than competitive prices. He argued that consumers did not have a range of choices about where they could go for health-care services; therefore, they relied on "blind faith" that nursing and medical care was of high quality and priced correctly. Finer elaborated on nursing as a specific " 'blind article' . . . the article itself is not blind but its various qualities and components are so subtle and complicated and the nature of demand so unpredictable that the traders [hospitals] may not be able to judge the price and the consumers will be even less able to detect whether they are being cheated."[197] In this situation, Finer argued, hospitals could "give services of a quality inferior to that which they would be compelled to render were they dependent for their solvency upon the retention of their customers in the face of lower prices and better services offered by a rival in the vicinity."[198]

While Finer and others criticized the virtual monopolistic position of hospitals, at the time little attention was drawn to the fact that physicians, rather than hospital administrators, controlled patient admissions to hospitals. Thus physicians actually controlled the cash flow in hospitals, thereby influencing hospital decisions toward medical priorities. This set of circumstances did not lead to emphasis on higher-quality nursing care. Instead, hospital and nursing administrators were consistently playing retroactive "catch-up" to rising demands for nurses to keep more beds and services open. More simply put, nursing care of the patients was an afterthought in a physician-centered, medical diagnoses-driven hospital system. It is little wonder that nursing underwent chronic hospital-led "shortages" throughout the period.

From 1946 until the mid-seventies Americans enthusiastically underwrote hospital-based care via voluntary health insurance, Medicare and Medicaid, and various other public and private programs which helped pay for care. Only in the latter seventies is there evidence of serious, widespread concern about the costs of the post-war decision to commit so much of our health-care resource on hospitals.

Contemporary public complaints about hospitals usually cite their high cost and access problems stemming from lack of insurance. But Americans now also recognize other limitations of hospital services. Over time, the custom of limiting hospital access and insurance payments to those people with medically treatable conditions in the acute-illness phase meant that chronically ill, aged, convalescent and otherwise dependent people had limited (or no) access to the most developed and best staffed institutions in our health-care system. And unfortunately, money to support alternatives such as home care or other community-based services, which could have substituted for hospital care, has been slow to follow those patients who were excluded because they do not qualify for hospital services.

The Work, Pay, and Education of Nurses

Since the patients for whom hospital nurses care are now being relocated to other settings, the future centrality of nursing to hospitals and hospitals to nursing is open to question. Just how will this historically important linkage change if the hospital becomes less central in our health-care system? Some nurses will follow their patients and re-direct their careers away from hospitals and toward community-based care. But how many, and just where will they practice?

Pressures to improve and expand nursing services in home care, nursing homes, and community clinics abound. For instance, Medicare expenditures for home-care services have exploded in recent years, growing from about 2 percent of the Medicare budget to more than 4 percent. This is still a small proportion of the total Medicare budget, but continued rapid increase will require a significant reallocation of resources. Evaluation of the outcomes of the 1982–7 Teaching Nursing Home Program suggests that adding geriatric nurse practitioners to nursing-home staffs can maximize patient care, reducing hospitalization and untoward complications. But the costs of placing master's-prepared nurses in nursing homes will require reallocating Medicare or other dollars from the hospital sector to long-term care.

A few nurses are starting to modify the health-care system by improving out-of-hospital services through systems such as community nursing centers. We will learn in the upcoming decade if nursing can summon the resources to improve community care, home-care services, and long-term care, as well as upgrade the quality of intensive nursing care in hospitals at the same time.

Shifting Loyalties

Three-quarters or more of all nurses practiced in hospitals during the second half of the twentieth century. That fact alone helps explain the historical merging of hospital and nursing interests and the difficulty of separating hospital and nursing policy. Nurses' dependence on hospitals and loyalty to the institutional ideal permeates nursing history. Moving nursing education into colleges and universities began to undermine nurses' loyalty to hospitals; relocating their patients to other care settings is now accelerating that trend.

The dichotomous nature of nurses' work, which includes both professionalized clinical care and social services, sustained confusion about who should and did do the work of nursing and exactly what constituted nursing work. Over time, nurses' work changed significantly, moving across geographic, professional and institutional boundaries. At the same time, studies repeatedly showed discrepancies in work practices among hospitals. This lack of a clear, shared description of nurses' work and lack of consensus on who should do it persists today. American nurses have a long history of responding to demands that they assume substantial responsibility for care of the sick with or without training and/or authority. This tendency was very pronounced during the period we studied; witness the invention of the intensive care nurse and the nurse practitioner.

Why were nurses given the burden of subsidizing the expansion of hospitals via their low wages for so many years? Why did they accept that task? One suggestion is that the tradition of trading work for training was a brilliant solution to the labor problems of women and the pre-insurance financial problems of hospitals. But the persistence of this pattern of low wages for caregivers for years after hospitals became solvent and then affluent is harder to justify. The custom of gender wage inequity, exploitation of lower-class and black entrants to the field, a large female labor supply, less than effective labor organizing by nurses, and the local control of wages by hospitals all contributed. In varying degrees most of these factors still influence the nursing field. Even when patients are relocated to other settings some form of nursing will still be needed. Should we not expect the nursing problems of the hospital era to spill over into other arenas of care?

The alternatives for practice now open to nurses are changing the background or context of the hospital–nursing negotiation. Now hospitals have to consider whether practice opportunities for nurses will expand outside their institutions to the degree that a new kind of hospital nursing shortage could emerge. That is, the next hospital nursing shortage could be due, not to rising demand from hospitals, but to competing demands from other sectors of the health-care system. Moreover, nurses will be unlikely to accept low wages to subsidize the financial problems of out-of-hospital care systems. The reluctance of nurses to move into nursing-home practice should be instructive in this regard.

Large health-care systems are attracting political support; in these systems hospitals are only a part, no longer the central player.[199] If this trend persists it is possible that, for the first time since the disappearance of private duty nursing, a truly competitive labor market for nursing could develop. Today, the most obvious indicator of this possible scenario is the ease with which home-care or visiting-nurse associations can recruit high quality nurses away from hospital practice.[200] On the other hand, this wage competition for nurses will be tempered by the extent to which large health-care systems come to dominate in any particular region. If a vertically organized health-care system controlled most of the nursing jobs in an area then it is more likely that a twenty-first-century version of the old monopsonistic control of nurses' salaries would ensue.

Although under the control of colleges, much of the clinical part of nursing education is still hospital-based. Moving nursing practice away from the hospital will demand significant change in patterns of nursing education. Many nurses rely on hospital employment and tuition subsidization through their employee benefits to help pay for advanced education after basic preparation. Converting to a more balanced health-care system which is less dependent on hospitals will set off a chain of consequences for educating and paying for the education of the next generations of nurses. Although many nurses pay for master's study out of their own pocket they will be deprived of easy access to weekend and part-time work.

Nurses Participating in Planning

New-found power among nurses is strikingly evident in any comparison between nurses' public behavior at the beginning and end of this forty-five-year history. The forcefulness and frequency with which nurses now participate in debates about their own field is in marked contrast to the 1940s and 1950s. Using the tools of economics and political science, research-based argument and informed journalism, as well as more traditional reminders of the essential work and social value of nurses, a wide spectrum of nursing voices is now heard. For the last decade or so nursing leaders have been unwilling to allow the field to be studied by economists, sociologists, physicians or administrators without equitable participation and leadership from nurses.

The women's movement and civil-rights movement made it much harder, though certainly not impossible, to continue to exclude nurses from negotiations both inside the health-care system and at policy levels in the public and private sectors. Better educated and more sophisticated nurses are at the conference table and arguing their case in the professional literature, the press, and the electronic media.

Many of the studies of nursing done in the last forty years may be criticized for their narrow focus on nursing in hospitals, and for neglecting the social context in which nursing and health care developed and operated. Indeed, many studies were not studies at all but simply polls of expert opinion. In another sense, however, the weaknesses of these studies, especially their predictive failures, testify to the excruciating difficulty of anticipating or predicting future events or even recognizing the system-wide implications of current decisions. Historian Rosemary Stevens argues that, since Americans lack an overall philosophy to give direction and co-herence, we are forced to assemble our policies as well as we can through negotiated consensus among shifting coalitions.[201] Forty years of nursing studies and their recommendations cannot be compared to any national goal since no real consensus on a national program ever was promulgated. Instead, what emerges from this retrospective review is serial response to constantly changing trends of belief and emphasis regarding hospital nursing. First, strategists relied on simply enlarging the supply of nurses; later, belief shifted to improving the skills of nurses through edu-cation and retention of more experienced nurses. Now, we see a trend toward de-institutionalization beginning to markedly alter the role, responsibility, and location of practice for nurses. Overall, however, Americans' preference for incrementalism and compro-mise tends to put off hard choices. During the hospital-nursing era that habit of procrastination helped sustain the idea that hospital nursing was permanently problematic.

Suggestions for the Future

Several recommendations related to nursing and to nurse–physician relationships are suggested by this review. First, it is crucial that nursing and medical practice and education issues are studied together. The rapid increases in the numbers of both nurses and physicians during the last 25 years (table 3.1), is the product of a series of expansionist decisions which need review.

Conclusions drawn about either profession in isolation from the other are necessarily incomplete and even misleading. We need to know how patients are cared for by doctors and nurses, evaluate the quality of services, and study provider and patient satisfaction.

Table 3.1 Active health manpower per 100,000 population, 1950–1992

Provider/year	1950	1960	1970	1980	1992
MD/100,000	144	144	158/143	190	230
RN/100,000	246	279	342/369	560	726

Source: United States Department of Health, Education, and Welfare (USDHEW), *Hearings of the Committee on Appropriations* (1973); National Center for Health Statistics, *Statistical Abstract of the United States, 1972*, p. 5; figures in bold are from US Health and Human Services, PHS, *Health, United States 1988* (DAHS Pub. No. 89-1232, 1988); Table 7, "Physician–Population Ratio," American Medical Association, *Socioeconomic Characteristics of Medical Practice 1994* (Center for Health Policy); USHHEW, Division of Nursing, *The Registered Nurse Population* (Washington DC: USGPO, 1992).

Exploring the distinct and overlapping work of doctors and nurses will clarify the knowledge needs and authority requirements of both professions. Such an examination must allow for the differences among hospitals, other care settings, patients and available care-givers. Urban areas versus rural communities, and community hospitals versus academic medical centers, are some examples of the delineations needed. Regionally focused studies would be most effective in terms of their potential applicability to our vast and heterogeneous health-care needs.

Many have suggested that medical and nursing education should strive to enhance the collaborative capabilities of each professional. The problem is that little usable information is at hand on the collective realities of medical and nursing practice or the impact of shared educational experiences; moreover, there are few rewards for faculty or students who seek to develop the latter. Nonetheless, isolationism among the health professions will have to be bridged.

We need to examine and evaluate the reallocation of clinical work between physicians and nurses and the allocation of new work to the two professions. We know that nurses and physicians are working together in new ways. Nurse practitioners with advanced skills are joining medical specialty practices to provide both nursing and general medical care to the patients in the practice. For instance, cardiovascular surgeons now employ such nurses to cope with the non-surgical and general health-care needs of their chronically ill patients. In some hospitals nurse practitioners carry out work formerly done by physicians in training, i.e. admission physicals, routine medical orders, clinical oversight, and communication with the patients attending physicians.[202]

For decades nurses in neonatal units and intensive care units have performed medical tasks; the same is true in inner-city clinics and rural health services. The 1980s' Teaching Nursing Home Project showed how frail, sick or demented patients in nursing homes can be assisted by skilled nurse clinicians linked to physicians by telephone. These reallocations of medical and nursing responsibility and new practice patterns are known through anecdotes and simple descriptions but not quantified. They need to be evaluated and, where appropriate, integrated in future planning in both medicine and nursing.[203]

This look at the recent past also highlights Americans' historical reluctance to admit and confront the actual high cost of nurse caretaking in hospitals. For all of the twentieth century hospitals developed and refined the role of safe substitute for family care for certain selected groups of patients. Hospitals, since World War II, have framed themselves in many ways: as centers of community care; as high-technology, life-saving institutions; and as corporate-style holding companies offering a complete horizon of cradle-to-grave health services. But, however the hospital presents itself, the burden of care it assumes is borne by the nurses who keep it constantly open. Hospitals are valued because of the medical services they provide, but needed because people using the services are too sick to care for themselves.

Clinging to the idea of a low-cost nurse while, at the same time, promising the best scientific, life-saving care is an American habit that history shows is the basis of much of the nursing problem. We need to distinguish the costs of nursing from other hospital charges so that informed choices can be made about the use of the nursing resource.

The cost of nursing, however well hidden, rose inexorably as we pursued a "do everything" medical agenda; the history of intensive care, for example, is grounded in a public and health-professional decision to ward off death at any cost. To succeed even some of the time, intensive care nurses must be very knowledgeable and experienced as well as numerous. Now, thirty or more years into the history of intensive care, thoughtful nurses and physicians who are directly involved in critical care are struggling to think in terms of doing less for at least some of the critically ill.[204] Considering the question of more judicious investment of nursing resources in the care of the critically ill immediately brings us to the other face of costly hospital nursing, which is our historic failure to ensure quality nurses for the sick outside of hospitals.

Hospitals, especially since the advent of prospective reimbursement, discharge people away from nursing care to their homes or other facilities. Nurses have not followed in the same proportions because the money to pay them was locked in the hospital sector of care. There is nothing new in this; the aged, the chronically ill, and those needing rehabilitation are expensive to care for and were systematically excluded as the curative twentieth-century mission of hospitals took hold.[205]

There is a permanent nursing shortage in nursing homes, for example, that society still chooses to tolerate. Even in the 1950s, when both the number and the quality of hospital nurses were low, nurses were not completely absent from hospitals. In present-day nursing homes nurses are truly scarce and those who are there are seriously over-committed and under-paid. We must reallocate some nursing resources to nursing homes unless we intend to consign patients who no longer qualify for acute hospital care to an unplanned, undebated reversal of a fifty-year promise of access to safe institutional care.

And, finally, the hospital nursing strategy that did work where it was tried and which still has value is the primary-nursing idea. It restored the concept of a specific nurse for each hospitalized patient that was lost when private duty nursing disappeared. As each patient's hospital stay grows shorter and more intense, pressure related to early, pre-ordained discharge falls on the primary nurse. Twenty-four-hour accountability and familiarity with each individual patient's situation are crucial to avoid serious error and abuse. The primary nurse monitors, detects changes, interprets and intervenes, supervises basic care and teaches his/her patients about their care.[206] Downsizing of hospital nursing staff creates an immediate threat to the primary-nursing system and invites failure in patient care.

Well-motivated and compassionate nursing care is both essential to humanistic hospital care and always threatened by cost pressures. The hospital nursing project of the next ten years will be to figure out how to effectively employ clinical nurse specialists with primary nurses and attending physicians to safely care for an ever more acutely ill hospital population. And to do that in a way that leaves some share of the health-care dollar for the majority of sick care which goes on outside the hospital.

Historians speak of the American hospital as an "institution through which the moral values of American society are expressed."[207] Over the forty-plus years since Americans decided to make the hospital the center of our health-care system the consequences of that decision emerged in unanticipated ways. Hospitals steadily increased their focus on intensive and short-term care, necessitating other ad hoc or institutional ways to care for those of the sick who did not qualify for hospital care. At the same time successful medical therapeutics and demographic changes shifted the weight of demands on the total care system away from short-term acute care. This accentuated the financial and health-worker imbalances created by over-investment in acute-care hospitals.

And inside the hospital, for many of the years since 1948, an "Upstairs, Downstairs" relationship persisted between "Downstairs" hospital nurses and "Upstairs" physicians and professional hospital administrators. Hospital expansion plans went forward assuming sufficient women workers would appear to make the institutions function. Both community hospitals and large academic medical centers became more elegant and expanded the volume and variety of services they offered. In spite of mushrooming technology these expanded services were, invariably, labor intensive. Planning for these institutions depended on an imagined supply of labor drawn from rural and lower middle-class or working-class women who, it was assumed, would always be there and would settle for an inexpensive education and a steady job.

Overlapping this scenario was a rapid escalation in the complexity of hospital nursing work which steadily made high-volume, low-cost nurse training more and more inadequate. And nurses increasingly resisted and resented their "Downstairs" role as they worked to make the hospital care system function. Nurses sought and obtained more education and began to control more aspects of care, as, for example, in intensive care and the various specialties. Relationships between nurses and hospitals and between nurses and physicians became more equitable and, at the same time, more filled with overt strains.

Nursing practice and nursing education, so deeply imbedded in hospitals, adapted to and made possible the intensification of hospital care. Now nurses will need to anticipate and plan for relocating more patient care outside of hospitals. Transformed since 1965, nursing continues to confront fundamental alterations in its role in the American health-care system. The largest of the health-care professions, it will be expected to produce a major proportion of direct health and sickness care both in and outside of institutions. How Americans and American nurses will respond to these insistent, ever changing demands is the story of the next generation.

Notes

1   In 1991 nursing salaries, which rose steeply for three years, leveled off but kept rising slowly. The average minimum annual salary for general nursing was $26,874; the average maximum salary was $40,194. "Nursing News," *RN* (September 1991): 13. In 1992 the national average salary reached $35,212. In 1993 starting pay in New York City averaged $40,000. Nurses in nursing homes did not benefit as much as hospital nurses; starting salaries averaged $3 an hour less for nursing home positions.

2   Cynthia Freund, Ph.D., Dean, School of Nursing, University of North Carolina, personal communication, September 1992.

3   Susan Reverby, *Ordered to Care: The Dilemma of American Nursing, 1850–1945* (Cambridge, MA: Cambridge University Press, 1987); Barbara Melosh, *The Physician's Hand: Work, Culture and Conflict in American Nursing* (Philadelphia: Temple University Press, 1982); Nancy Tomes, "'A Little World of Their Own': The Pennsylvania Hospital Training School for Nurses," *Journal of the History of Medicine and Allied Sciences*, 33 (1978): 507–30; Celia Davis (ed.), *Rewriting Nursing History* (Totowa, NJ: Barnes and Noble Books, 1980).

4   Charles E. Rosenberg, *The Care of Strangers: The Rise of America's Hospital System* (New York: Basic Books, 1987). Morris Vogel, *The Invention of the Modern Hospital: Boston 1870–1930* (Chicago: University of Chicago Press, 1980). David Rosner, *A Once Charitable Enterprise: Hospitals and Health Care in Brooklyn and New York, 1885–1915* (Princeton, NJ: Princeton University Press, 1982). Rosemary Stevens, *In Sickness and in Wealth: American Hospitals in the Twentieth Century* (New York: Basic Books, 1989). Diana Elizabeth Long and Janet Golden (eds), *The American General Hospital: Communities and Social Contexts* (Ithaca and London: Cornell University Press, 1989).

5   Reverby, *Ordered to Care*: p. 79. For an in-depth discussion of the transition from private duty to hospital staff nursing, see Marilyn E. Flood, "The Troubling Expedient: General Staff Nursing in United States Hospitals in the 1930s, a Means to Institutional, Educational, and Personal Ends" (Ph.D. dissertation, University of California, Berkeley, 1981).

6   Darlene Clark Hine, *Black Women in White: Racial Conflict and Cooperation in the Nursing Profession, 1890–1950* (Bloomington: Indiana University Press, 1989) p. 188. By 1960, 6.5 percent of the total RN workforce was nonwhite, US Department HEW, Division of Nursing, *Source Book: Nursing Personnel*, DHEW Publication No. 75–43 (Washington DC: US Government Printing Office, 1973): 30.

7   Stevens, *In Sickness and in Wealth*, p. 203. Stevens notes that infectious disease struck the poor more often, while chronic illnesses were the lot of the longer-lived affluent.

8   US Department of Commerce, Bureau of the Census, *Historical Statistics of the United States – Colonial Times to 1970*, Part I (Washington DC: US Government Printing Office, 1975) p. 55.

9   "Hospital Beds in the United States," *Public Health Reports*, 67 (March 1952): 313.

10   Paul Starr, *The Social Transformation of American Medicine* (New York: Basic Books, 1982), see especially Book Two, chapter 2. Also Julie Fairman, "New Hospitals, New Nurses, New Spaces: The Development of Intensive Care Units, 1950–1965" (Ph.D. dissertation, University of Pennsylvania, 1992) p. 31.

11   Fairman, "New Hospitals, New Nurses."

12   Lucille Petry Leone, interview by Joan Lynaugh, 11 November 1989. Leone was nurse consultant to the United States Public Health Service (USPHS) from 1942 until she became Chief of its Nursing Division in the late 1940s. Parran's comment was a response to her wartime recommendation that the USPHS Cadet Nurse program favor "good" nursing schools by giving its educational subsidies to students enrolling in higher-quality programs.

13   Much has been written about the peculiar nursing education system. An excellent account of the nursing situation is Anselm Strauss, "The Structure and Ideology of American Nursing," in Fred Davis (ed.), *The Nursing Profession* (New York: John Wiley and Sons, 1966) pp. 60–108. See especially pp. 70–2. Historians took up the task of interpreting the story with Melosh's *The Physician's Hand* (1982) and Reverby's *Ordered to Care* (1987).

14   Isabel Stewart, "A Guide for the Organization of Collegiate Schools of Nursing" (National Nursing Council for War Service and the Association of Collegiate Schools of Nursing: 1790 Broadway, NYC, 1942). Stewart carefully laid out a plan for better training of nurses but college-based programs developed very slowly. The Hospital Survey and Reconstruction Act (Hill Burton) was a watershed event

in both hospital and nursing history. By 1949, 42 states reported construction under way. Hill Burton was followed by a steady flow of expansionist amendments (1954, 1956, 1958, 1961, 1964, 1970) until 1972. By 1971, $13 billion (3.7 billion in federal dollars) had been spent.

15 Fred J. Cook, *The Plot Against the Patient* (Englewood Cliffs, NJ: Prentice-Hall, 1962) p. 164.

16 Susan Reverby discusses this relationship more explicitly in "The Search for the Hospital Yardstick: Nursing and the Rationalization of Hospital Work," pp. 206–25, in Susan Reverby and David Rosner (eds), *Health Care in America: Essays in Social History* (Philadelphia: Temple University Press, 1979).

17 Margaret Bridgeman, *Collegiate Education for Nursing* (New York: Russell Sage Foundation, 1953) p. 11.

18 For further discussion, see Barbara L. Brush, "Shortage as Shorthand for the Crisis in Caring," *Nursing and Health Care*, 13 (November 1992): 480–6. Despite increases in registered nurses from 90,746 to 130,838 (full-time) and from 17,188 to 77,359 (part-time) between 1948 and 1962, debate continuously focused on the shortage of nursing personnel.

19 Brush, "Shortage as Shorthand," pp. 480–6. Actually, due to the rapid growth and diversification of hospitals in this period, the numerical and deployment problems in nursing were of the hospitals' own creation. Funding for hospital expansion did not provide dollars for essential caregivers.

20 Mary Roberts, *American Nursing, History and Interpretation* (New York: Macmillan, 1954) p. 472.

21 Esther Lucile Brown, *Nursing for the Future: A Report Prepared for the National Nursing Council* (New York: Russell Sage Foundation, 1948) p. 7.

22 Eli Ginzberg, *A Program for the Nursing Profession by the Committee on the Function of Nursing* (New York: Macmillan, 1948) p. 2.

23 American Medical Association, "Report of the Committee on Nursing Problems," *JAMA*, 137 (October 1948): 878; "Progress of the ANA's Older Nurse Project," *American Journal of Nursing*, 53 (September 1953): 1101.

24 Ferdinand Lundberg and Marynia F. Farnham, *Modern Women: The Lost Sex* (New York: Harper and Brothers, 1947) p. 368.

25 See Lyndia Flanagan's account of the American Nurses' Association in this period, in *Brave New Frontiers: ANA's Economic and General Welfare Program, 1946–1986* (American Nurses' Association, 1984).

26 Lily Mary David, "The Economic Status of the Nursing Profession," *American Journal of Nursing*, 47 (July 1947): 458.

27 Lily Mary David "Economic Status of Private Duty and General Staff Nurses," *American Journal of Nursing*, 47 (October 1947): 671.

28 Fairman, "New Hospitals, New Nurses," p. 106. The PNA

recommended average monthly salaries of $300 in 1958 and $365 in 1962, Chestnut Hill Hospital offered $300 in 1959 and $315 in 1962, and the Hospital of the University of Pennsylvania $260 and $320 respectively. For more on nurses' wages see Pamela Frances Cipriano, "Compensation of Staff Nurses Employed in United States Hospitals from 1960 to 1990" (Ph.D. dissertation, University of Utah, 1992).

29   Donald Yett, "The Supply of Nurses: An Economist's View," *Hospital Progress*, 46 (February 1965): 99.

30   United States Census Bureau, *1960 Census of Population: Characteristics of the Population*, Part I, table 201.

31   "Letters Pro and Con," *American Journal of Nursing* (October 1955): 1156.

32   US Department HEW, *Source Book, Nursing Personnel*, DHEW Publication No. 75–43 (Bethesda, MD: US Government Printing Office, 1974): 35.

33   Ginzberg, *A Program for the Nursing Profession*, p. 15.

34   Ibid., p. 47.

35   Brown, *Nursing for the Future*, p. 63.

36   Ibid., p. 62.

37   For further discussion, see Monte Calvert, *The Mechanical Engineer in America, 1830–1910* (Baltimore: Johns Hopkins Press, 1967).

38   David, "The Economic Status of the Nursing Profession," p. 461.

39   Ginzberg, *A Program for the Nursing Profession*, p. 34.

40   Florence Nightingale, *Notes on Nursing: What It Is and What It Is Not* (Reprint Edition; New York: Dover Publications, 1969). Nightingale and her successors emphasized the importance of creating and maintaining a healthful atmosphere to "put the patient in the best condition for nature to heal him."

41   Eleanor C. Lambertsen, *Nursing Team Organization and Functioning* (New York: Teacher's College, Columbia University, 1953) p. iii.

42   Isabel Maitland Stewart, *The Education of Nurses: Historical Foundations and Modern Trends* (New York: Macmillan, 1943) p. 149. Stewart notes that adoption of the efficiency movement by some hospitals and nursing leaders was an attempt to deal with rapid technological change.

43   Reverby, "Search for the Hospital Yardstick," p. 215.

44   Frances L. George and Ruth P. Kuehn, *Patterns of Patient Care: Some Studies of the Utilization of Nursing Service Personnel* (New York: Macmillan, 1955) p. 57.

45   Ginzberg, *A Program for the Nursing Profession*, p. 55.

46   Ibid., p. 105.

47   William K. Miller, "An Unfair Burden for 1100 Hospitals," *Hospitals, JAHA*, 33 (1 October 1959): 42.

48   Ibid., p. 42. Miller's statistics were based on a cost-analysis study by Scovell, Wellington & Company, Boston, Massachusetts.

49   US Department of Health, Education, and Welfare, *Toward Quality in Nursing: Needs and Goals* (Washington DC: USGPO, 1963) p. 10. See Mildred Montag, *Community College Education for Nursing: An Experiment in Technical Education for Nursing* (New York: McGraw Hill, 1959) for the original ADN concept. It was intended to prepare nurse technicians to work under the direction of nurses prepared at the baccalaureate level.

50   National Commission on Community Health Services, National Task Forces Project, *Health Manpower: Action to Meet Community Needs* (Washington DC: Public Affairs Press, 1967) p. 52; Nona Y. Glazer, "Between a Rock and a Hard Place: Women's Professional Organizations in Nursing, and Class, Racial, and Ethnic Inequalities," 5 (September 1991): 351–72. This trend continues today. Over 22 percent of graduates from LPN programs in 1989 were minorities, compared with 16.3 percent of RN graduates. See NLN Division of Research. *Nursing DataSource 1992*, Volume I (New York: NLN Press, 1993) p. 15.

51   US Department HEW, *Source Book: Nursing Personnel*, p. 30.

52   David Barton Smith, "The Racial Integration of Medical and Nursing Associations in the United States," *Hospital and Health Services Administration*, 8, unpublished manuscript. See also Darlene Clark Hine, *Black Women in White*.

53   Smith, "The Racial Integration," p. 9. See R. Cunningham, "Jim Crow M.D.," *The Nation* (7 June 1952): 548–51.

54   See Darlene Hine, *Black Women in White*, for fuller discussion.

55   Barbara L. Brush, "'Exchangees' or Employees?: The Exchange Visitor Program and Foreign Nurse Immigration to the United States, 1945–1990," *Nursing History Review*, 1 (1993): 171–80. Brush argues that the EVP became an inexpensive recruiting mechanism for short-staffed hospitals.

56   Marthe Jean Broadhurst, *Nurses from Abroad: Values in International Exchange of Persons* (New York: American Nurses' Foundation, 1962). Broadhurst's study is the only detailed account of the EVP and its participants. She interviewed and recorded the experiences of 60 graduate nurses from 15 countries who arrived under the EVP between 1956 and 1961.

57   Fairman, "New Hospitals, New Nurses," p. 11.

58   Ibid., p. 39.

59   Jack C. Haldeman and Faye G. Abdellah, "Concepts of Progressive Patient Care," *Hospitals*, 33 (16 May 1959): 38–42. *W. K. Kellogg Foundation: The First Half Century, 1930–1980 – Private Approaches to Public Needs* (Battle Creek, MI: W. K. Kellogg Foundation, 1980) p. 61.

60   Haldeman and Abdellah, "Concepts."

61   Ibid., p. 40.

62   For the best historical analysis of the implications of various hospital

designs over time, see John D. Thompson and Grace Goldin, *The Hospital: A Social and Architectural History* (New Haven and London: Yale University Press, 1975). John D. Thompson later was one of the architects of the concept of diagnostic-related groups as a device for pre-payment for hospital care.

63   The American Association of Critical-Care Nurses, founded in 1969 as the American Association of Cardiovascular Nurses, was a direct result of nurses' efforts to educate themselves for new intensive care unit patient demands.

64   Herman Finer, *Administration and the Nursing Services* (New York: Macmillan, 1952) p. vii.

65   Ibid., p. 145.

66   Ibid.

67   Henry T. Maschal, "Developing the Nursing Service Budget," *Hospital Management*, 75 (January 1953): 64–71, 76 and 77, 94. Part of this economical approach was to make sure that head nurses knew the costs of linens, bandages and other supplies used by staff nurses and ensured that they were used properly.

68   Finer, *Administration*, p. 317.

69   Reverby, *Ordered to Care*, p. 121.

70   Ibid., p. 124. Also, see Ruth Sleeper, "A Reaffirmation of Belief in the Diploma School," *Nursing Outlook*, 6 (November 1958): 616–18, to sample a negative view of change shared by some nurse leaders. Sleeper argued that the value of keeping hospital beds open to the public overrode the profession's call for upgrading education for nurses.

71   Reverby, *Ordered to Care*, p. 190.

72   Hans Mauksch, "The Organizational Context of Nursing Practice," in Fred Davis (ed.), *The Nursing Profession: Five Sociological Essays* (New York: John Wiley & Sons, 1966) pp. 109–37.

73   Everett C. Hughes, Helen McGill and Irwin Deutscher, *Twenty Thousand Nurses Tell their Story: A Report on Studies of Nursing Functions Sponsored by the ANA* (Philadelphia: J. B. Lippincott, 1958) p. 139.

74   Hilda M. Torrop, "Today's Practical Nurse: Concepts Behind her Education," *Hospitals, JAHA*, 33 (16 August 1959): 46.

75   "Letters Pro and Con," *American Journal of Nursing* (March 1950): 8, and (December 1949): 6.

76   Fairman, "New Hospitals, New Nurses," p. 108.

77   Ibid., p 108.

78   "Research and the ANA Program for Studies of Nursing Functions," *American Journal of Nursing*, 50 (December 1950): 767–70.

79   Hughes, McGill, and Deutscher, *Twenty Thousand Nurses*, p. 124.

80   Ibid., p. 131.

81   Faye G. Abdellah and Eugene Levine, "Work-sampling Applied to the Study of Nursing Personnel," *Nursing Research*, 3 (January 1954).

82   Thomas R. Ford and Diane D. Stephenson, *Institutional Nurses: Roles,*

Relationships and Attitudes in Three Alabama Hospitals (Alabama: University of Alabama Press, 1954).

83   The Government Research Center, University of Kansas, *The Study of Activities of Registered Professional Nurses in Small Kansas Hospitals,* prepared for the Kansas Nurses' Association, 1953. They noted that RNs on the 11 p.m.–7 a.m. shift did the bulk of paperwork activity including writing up charts, transferring MDs' orders to Kardexs and making up medicine cards.

84   Hughes et al., *Twenty Thousand Nurses,* p. 147.

85   Genevieve Meyer, *Tenderness and Technique: Nursing Values in Transition* (Los Angeles: Institute of Industrial Relations, University of California, 1960) p. 9.

86   Phoebe H. Gordon, "Who Does What – The Report of a Nursing Activities Study," *American Journal of Nursing,* 53 (May 1953): 564–6. The study was conducted at the Charles T. Miller Hospital in St Paul, Minnesota.

87   Donald D. Stewart, *The Function of the General-Duty Nurse in Ten Arkansas Hospitals: A Progress Report to the Arkansas State Nurses' Association,* 15 August 1954.

88   For further comparison among surveys, see Louis J. Kroeger and Associates, *Nursing Practice in California Hospitals: A Report Based on a Study of Actual Practice in 40 California Hospitals* (California Nurses' Association, 1953); Division of Nursing Resources, Public Health Service, US Department of HEW, *For Better Nursing in Michigan: A Survey of Needs and Resources* (Detroit, MI: Cunningham Drug Company Foundation, 1954); Governmental Research Center, University of Kansas, *A Study of the Activities of Registered Professional Nurses in Small Kansas Hospitals* (Kansas State Nurses' Association, 1953); Joint Committee on Nursing Services of the Washington State Nurses' Association and the Washington State Leagues of Nursing Education, *Report of Nursing Functions Study: An Analysis of the Nursing Activities of a Medical Service in Two Urban Hospitals and the Combined Medical Surgical Service of a Small Community Hospital in the State of Washington* (Washington Nurses' Association, 1953).

89   Herman Finer, arguing in his widely read essay on nursing administration *Administration and the Nursing Services* (New York: Macmillan, 1952), pp. 116–29.

90   Brush, in "Shortage as Shorthand," calls for a wider analysis including nonrational factors to improve predictive success when considering nursing shortages.

91   George and Kuehn, *Patterns of Patient Care,* pp. 2, 3.

92   An important exception to this was the segment of the hospital system owned and operated by nursing sisters and the Roman Catholic Church. The internal working and relationships of these institutions are only now beginning to attract historians' attention. See, for example, Kathleen M. Joyce, "Science and the Saints:

American Catholics and Health Care, 1880–1930" (Ph.D. dissertation, Princeton University, 1995).

93   David, "Economic Status of Private Duty and General Staff Nurses," p. 671.

94   United States Census Bureau, *1960 Census of Population: Characteristics of the Population*, Part I, table 201.

95   Meyer, *Tenderness and Technique*.

96   By the 1970s hospital leaders began to act as though they agreed with Meyer, *Tenderness and Technique*, as they replaced lesser-trained LPNs and aides with more and more registered nurses who required little supervision.

97   National Institute of Health, *Health Manpower Source Book 21: Allied Health Manpower Supply and Requirements, 1950–1980* (Washington DC: US Government Printing Office, 1970).

98   The population of the United States grew from 151,325,798 in 1950 to 203,302,031 in 1970. *The World Almanac 1992* (New York: World Almanac, 1992) p. 75. The number of physicians grew slowly until 1970. Between 1950 and 1960, the number grew by about 10 percent; then in the years between 1970 and 1986, the number of physicians jumped from 143 per 100,000 to 218 per 100,000. US Health and Human Services, Public Health Service, *Health, United States 1988* (DAHS Pub. No. 89–1232, 1988).

99   Odin Anderson, *Toward an Unambiguous Profession: A Review of Nursing*, pamphlet (Chicago, IL: Center for Health Administration Studies, 1968): 16, 26. Data about nursing personnel vary greatly from study to study. Sometimes the number of hospital nurses is confounded with the number of nurses in the hospital's school of nursing; sometimes not. It is often difficult to tell whether statistical reports select out part-time nurses from full-time. We have tried to use numbers that make sense, but we are in sympathy with Flint and Spensley who complained, " . . . there are very many data about nursing personnel, but very little [reliable] information, . . . to resolve uncertainty." Robert Flint and Karen Spensley, "Recent Issues in Nursing Manpower: A Review," *Nursing Research*, 18 (June 1969): 217–29.

100 Nursing had been the only health profession to come out in support of Medicare and Medicaid prior to their enactment.

101 John D. Stoeckle, "The Citadel Cannot Hold: Technologies Go Outside the Hospital, Patients and Doctors Too," *Milbank Quarterly*, 73 (1995): 3–17. Stoeckle cites the decline in bedrest as a therapeutic strategy for a variety of acute and chronic problems as a factor in reducing hospital use.

102 The issues of 1970s nursing are very successfully analyzed in Michael Millman (ed.), *Nursing Personnel and the Changing Health Care System* (Cambridge, MA: Ballinger, 1978), which reports the proceedings of a nursing conference sponsored by the Conservation of Human

Resources [institute] at Columbia University in New York, held at Harrison House, Glen Cove, Long Island, in 1977.

103   Frances Reiter, "The Nurse-Clinician," *American Journal of Nursing*, 66 (February 1966): 274–80. Faye Abdellah and Eugene Levine reporting in *Nursing Outlook*, 3 (June 1954): 15.

104   Anderson, *Toward an Unambiguous Profession*, pp. 10–12. See also Elmina Mary Price, *Learning Needs of Registered Nurses* (New York: Teachers College Press, 1967), for a discouraging portrait of nurses' own evaluation of their abilities to meet patient care problems.

105   Doris Schwartz, "Some Thoughts on Quality in Nursing Service," *International Nursing Review*, 14 (March/April 1967): 29.

106   *Report of the National Advisory Commission on Health Manpower*, vol. 1 (Washington DC: US Government Printing Office, 1967) p. 23. Lyndon Johnson appointed this group of business leaders, physicians, and staff from philanthropic organizations. The Commission did its work through several panels of experts. One nurse was named among the 83 participants.

107   See the report of the 1983 Committee on Nursing and Nursing Education of the Institute of Medicine, for language and reasoning essentially similar to that of the National Advisory Commission.

108   This dilemma is well developed by Patricia Prescott in a recent essay, P. Prescott, "The Nurse Labor Market: Considerations for the 1990s," in *Charting Nursing's Future*, ed. Linda Aiken and Claire Fagin (Philadelphia: J. B. Lippincott, 1992) pp. 40–59.

109   See, for example, Committee on the Grading of Nursing Schools [Director: May Ayres Burgess], *Nursing Schools Today and Tomorrow* (New York City: n.p., 1934).

110   Report of the National Advisory Commission, p. 30. Dr Rozella Schlotfeldt, Dean of the School of Nursing at Western Reserve University, was the lone nurse on the Commission panels – she was on the Education and Supply Panel. In 1969 she led the second effort to "unify" nursing education and nursing services at a major medical center. The first such demonstration was launched in 1956 by Dean Dorothy Smith at the University of Florida at Gainesville.

111   Anderson, *Toward an Unambiguous Profession*, p. 12.

112   Frances Reiter and Marguerite Kakosh, "Quality of Nursing Care – A Report of a Field-Study to Establish Criteria," typescript (New York: Graduate School of Nursing, New York Medical College, March 1963). So far we have not been able to discover why this study was not published when completed in 1954.

113   Laurie M. Gunter, "Some Problems in Nursing Care and Services," in Bonnie Bullough and Vern Bullough (eds), *Issues in Nursing – Selected Readings* (New York: Springer, 1966) pp. 152–6. This paper lays out the practice–education issues as seen by an experienced nurse educator of the time.

114   Some estimates suggest the number of active private duty nurses fell

by more than 40 percent during World War II. Mary Roberts, *American Nursing: History and Interpretation* (New York: Macmillan, 1954) p. 363.

115 Vicki Wilson, "From Sentinels to Specialists," *American Journal of Nursing*, 90 (October 1990): 33. Aramine was a drug used at the time to elevate low blood pressure in instances of shock.

116 Progressive Patient Care is discussed in greater detail in chapter 1.

117 Rose Laub Coser, *Life in the Ward* (East Lansing, MI: Michigan State University Press, 1962). Coser's study described and analyzed the social role of the patient in a ward of a general hospital, institutional behavior patterns and value systems that prevailed in the ward, and relationships that developed among patients and between patients and staff.

118 Leonard Stein, "The Doctor–Nurse Game," *Archives of General Psychiatry*, 16 (1967): 699–703. Twenty-three years later Stein and two medical colleagues revisited the topic, outlining the more egalitarian, interdependent relationships between physicians and nurses that had evolved in the intervening years but acknowledging the continuing problems of competition and discomfort between the two professions. Leonard Stein et al., "The Doctor–Nurse Game Revisited," *New England Journal of Medicine*, 322 (22 February 1990): 546–9.

119 See, for instance, Anderson, *Toward an Unambiguous Profession*, pp. 12 and 23; Anselm Strauss, "The Structure and Ideology of American Nursing: An Interpretation," in Fred Davis (ed.), *The Nursing Profession* (New York: John Wiley and Sons, 1966) pp. 60–108. In the 1970s Barbara Bates, a physician, inserted this theme into the mainstream medical literature, see B. Bates, "Doctor and Nurse: Changing Roles and Relations," *New England Journal of Medicine*, 283 (16 July 1970): 129–34, and B. Bates, "Physician and Nurse Practitioner: Conflict and Reward," *Annals of Internal Medicine*, 82 (May 1975): 702–6. For an historical overview of nurse–physician relations see Joan E. Lynaugh, "Narrow Passageways: Nurses and Physicians in Conflict and Concert since 1875," in *The Physician as Captain of the Ship: A Critical Reappraisal* (Dordrecht and Boston: D. Reidel Publishing, 1988) pp. 23–37.

120 There is a substantial literature and debate about the matter of "professional dominance." Among others, Marie Haug has argued that there is a general decline in the knowledge monopoly of physicians because of better public education, rejection of medical authority, and, more recently, broad access to knowledge through computers. In the instance of nursing, sharing of knowledge was forced by pressures to increase access to valued medical services. The physician gatekeeper both stepped and was pushed out of the way. See, for Haug, Wolinsky and other viewpoints on professional dominance, Marie R. Haug, "A Re-examination of the Hypothesis of

Physician Deprofessionalization," and others in "The Changing Character of the Medical Profession," *Milbank Quarterly, Supplement 2*, 66 (1988).

121 Joan E. Lynaugh and Julie Fairman, "New Nurses, New Spaces: A Preview of the AACN History Study," *American Journal of Critical Care*, 1 (July 1992): 21.

122 Barbara Rollins, RN, Springdale, Arkansas [telephone interview by Joan Lynaugh], March 1990.

123 Rosemary Stevens, *In Sickness and In Wealth*, p. 296.

124 Daniel M. Fox, *Power and Illness: The Failure and Future of American Health Policy* (Berkeley: University of California Press, 1993). In his critique of American health policy priorities Fox argues that over-investment in care of acute illnesses and lack of resources committed to prevention and care of chronic illnesses has plagued American health planning for 75 years.

125 Florence E. Dunn and Miriam G. Shupp, "The Recovery Room – A Wartime Economy," *American Journal of Nursing*, 43 (March 1943): 279–81. Decisions about using precious space, and cooperation among administration, nursing and medicine were motivated by the difficult problems of staffing regular hospital wards to care for post-operative patients during World War II.

126 Marie Manthey et al., "Primary Nursing: A Return to the Concept of 'My Nurse' and 'My Patient'," *Nursing Forum*, 9 (January 1970): 65–84.

127 A thoughtful analysis of primary nursing and team nursing as well as a useful bibliography of studies and commentary is found in Kathryn G. Gardner, *The Effects of Primary Versus Team Nursing on Quality of Patient Care and Impact on Nursing Staff and Costs – A Five Year Study* (Rochester, NY: Rochester General Hospital, 1989). The study was funded by The Pew Charitable Trusts.

128 Joyce Clifford, "Professional Nursing Practice in a Hospital Setting," in Linda H. Aiken and Susan Gortner (eds), *Nursing in the 1980s: Crises, Opportunities, Challenges* (Philadelphia: J. B. Lippincott, 1982); and Mitchell T. Rabkin, "The Hospital as a Social System," *Transactions and Studies of the College of Physicians of Philadelphia*, XII (June 1990): 207–25.

129 Luther Christman, "A Microanalysis of the Nursing Division of One Medical Center," in Michael Millman (ed.), *Nursing Personnel and the Changing Health Care System* (Cambridge, MA: Ballinger, 1978) pp. 133, 151.

130 The Secretary's Committee to Study Extended Roles for Nurses, *Extending the Scope of Nursing Practice* (Washington DC: Government Printing Office, 1971).

131 "Medicine and Nursing in the 1970s: Position Statement," *Journal of the American Medical Association*, 213 (14 September 1970): 1881–3.

132 Henry Silver, Loretta Ford, and Lewis Day, "The Pediatric Nurse

Practitioner Program," *Journal of the American Medical Association*, 204 (22 April, 1968): 88–92.

133   Loretta C. Ford, "Myths and Misconceptions Re the Nurse Practitioner," *Critical Issues in Nursing in the Twentieth Century*, (Tarrytown, NY: Rockefeller Archive Center, 20 and 21 May 1993).

134   Unpublished Board information materials (1973), Archives, W. K. Kellogg Foundation, Battle Creek, MI. The Foundation invested about $1.5 million in the National Joint Practice Commission during the 1970s.

135   Susan Gortner, "Commentary," in Linda Aiken and Susan Gortner (eds), *Nursing in the 1980s – Crisis, Opportunities, Challenges* (Philadelphia: J. B. Lippincott, 1982) p. 499.

136   Results are in Harry A. Sultz et al., *Longitudinal Study of Nurse Practitioners, Phases I, II, and III* (all published by the US Government Printing Office and dated 1976, 1978, and 1980).

137   *Higher Education for American Democracy: A Report of the President's Commission on Higher Education* (Washington DC: US Government Printing Office, 1947). This report is usually called the "Truman Report."

138   Mildred L. Montag, *Community College Education for Nursing* (New York: McGraw-Hill, 1959); and Bernice Anderson, *Nursing Education in Community Junior Colleges* (Philadelphia: J. B. Lippincott, 1966). For a critique of the community college, see Steven Brint and Jerome Karabel, *The Diverted Dream: Community Colleges and the Promise of Educational Opportunity in America, 1900–1985* (New York and Oxford: Oxford University Press, 1989).

139   American Nurses' Association, *Educational Preparation for Nurse Practitioners and Assistants to Nurses: A Position Paper* (American Nurses' Association, 1965).

140   *An Abstract for Action*, ed. Jerome P. Lysaught, National Commission for the Study of Nursing and Nursing Education (New York: McGraw-Hill, 1970) pp. 81–147.

141   *Abstract for Action*, p. 40.

142   Elizabeth Bear, Ph.D., RN, "Oral History of Dr Esther Lucile Brown," Tape no. 1 (Ph.D. dissertation, University of Texas at Austin, 1986).

143   Kenneth Ludmerer discusses the consensus that developed between the academic elite and medical practitioners on the improvement of medical education at the turn of the twentieth century. K. Ludmerer, *Learning to Heal: The Development of American Medical Education* (New York: Basic Books, 1985) pp. 166–97.

144   Esther Lucile Brown, a sociologist, tracked and reported on nursing throughout her 40-year career. Author of a series of studies of American nursing, she also headed a group of sociologists based at the Russell Sage Foundation who analyzed the "nursing problem" in the 1960s. Brown's studies include: *Nursing for the Future* (New York: Russell Sage Foundation, 1948); *Newer Dimensions of Patient Care, Parts*

1, 2, and 3 (New York: Russell Sage Foundation, 1965); and *Nursing Reconsidered – A study of Change, Parts 1 and 2* (Philadelphia: J. B. Lippincott, 1971). The interview with Dr Brown was conducted just a few years before her death in 1991.

145 Bear, "Oral History," Tape no. 1.

146 Department of Health, Education and Welfare, *Progress Report on Nurse Training, 1970: Report to the President and the Congress* (Washington DC: US Government Printing Office, 1970).

147 Uwe Reinhardt, "Nursing Personnel in the Context of Health Manpower Policy," in Michael Millman (ed.), *Nursing Personnel and the Changing Health Care System* (Cambridge, MA: Ballinger, 1978) p. 17.

148 Bernard Bloom and Osler Peterson, "Physician Manpower Expansionism: A Policy Review," *Annals of Internal Medicine,* 90 (February 1979): 249–56.

149 "Nursing Capitation Grants: A Ten Year Summary" (Center for the Study of the History of Nursing, unpublished typescript, 1981).

150 Joan Lynaugh, "Philanthropy and American Nursing: The Case of the W. K. Kellogg Foundation 1930–1980," unpublished manuscript, 1996.

151 Eli Ginzberg does not comment on social equity in his earliest report on nursing, *A Program for the Nursing Profession* (1948), but later, in the 1970s, he suggests that accepting the baccalaureate standard for entry would be a direct assault on social mobility goals. See Eli Ginzberg, "Policy Directions," in M. Millman, *Nursing Personnel and the Changing Health Care System* (Cambridge, MA: Ballinger, 1978). In the 1980s, addressing nursing shortage, Ginzberg assumes that blacks can only enter nursing through two-year programs. Eli Ginzberg, "Nurses for the Future – Facing the Facts and Figures," *American Journal of Nursing* (Supplement) (December 1987): 1588–600.

152 Ginzberg, "Policy Directions," p. 271.

153 As of 1991 about 15 percent of nursing graduates were nonwhite: 11.1 percent black, 3.2 percent Hispanic, 3.0 percent Asian, and 0.6 percent American Indian. Baccalaureate programs in historically black colleges now number about 30; the first successful program was opened at Florida A&M University in 1936. Baccalaureate programs report the largest percentage of minority students with the exception of American Indians. Of 18,571 baccalaureate graduates in 1990, 1,910 were African American, *Nursing DataSource, 1991: Volume 1, Trends in Contemporary Nursing Education* (New York: National League for Nursing, 1991) pp. 5, 70.

154 Minority enrollment in programs leading to professional nursing ranged from 17.24 percent to 15.4 percent in 1990, 1991, and 1992. The largest proportion chose baccalaureate programs, then associate-degree, and last hospital-based diploma programs. *Nursing*

DataSource, 1993: Volume 1 (New York: National League for Nursing, 1993).

155   See Carrie Lenburg (ed.), *Open Learning and Career Mobility in Nursing* (Saint Louis: C. V. Mosby, 1975), for a collection of papers on this topic. Open admissions policies in two- and four-year colleges created severe problems for nurse educators, who had to develop a certain and reliable standard of technical proficiency in their students before granting degrees.

156   Millman, *Nursing Personnel in the Changing Health Care System*, p. 257.

157   In 1953 the mean annual salary (adjusted for inflation) was $3,324; in 1973 it was $6,396. This was an improvement; the effect of inflation, however, curtailed advances in real buying power. By 1989, in response to severe shortage, the average annual salary rose to $28,834. Salaries continued to rise at a slower pace; by 1993 starting pay in New York City averaged about $40,000.

158   American Nurses' Association, "The Nation's Nurses," 1972 Inventory of Registered Nurses (American Nurses' Association, 1974).

159   For a dissenting voice regarding baccalaureate education as the entry point, see Myrtle Adelotte, "Nursing Education: Shaping the Future," in *Charting Nursing's Future*, ed. Linda Aiken and Claire Fagin (Philadelphia: J. B. Lippincott, 1992) pp. 462–84. We are grateful to Rozella Scholdtfeldt, Dean Emeritus at Frances Payne Bolton School of Nursing, Case Western Reserve University, Cleveland, Ohio, for providing insight regarding the links between advanced nursing practice and baccalaureate improvements in the 1970s.

160   Mathy D. Mezey and Joan E. Lynaugh, "The Teaching Nursing Home Program – Outcomes of Care," *Nursing Clinics of North America*, 24 (September 1989): 769–80.

161   Bonnie Bullough, "Alternative Models for Specialty Nursing Practice," *Nursing and Health Care*, 13 (May 1992): 255.

162   George Rosen, *The Specialization of Medicine* (New York: Froben Press, 1944; Reprint Edition, Arno Press, 1972) p. 14.

163   See Donna Zschoche and Lillian E. Brown, "Intensive Care Nursing: Specialism, Junior Doctoring, or Just Nursing?" *American Journal of Nursing*, 69 (November 1969): 2370–4, for one of the earliest accounts of nurses' expanded roles in "intensive care."

164   Linda Aiken, "Charting the Future of Hospital Nursing," *Image: Journal of Nursing Scholarship*, 22 (Spring 1990): 72–8.

165   Shirley A. Smoyak, "Specialization in Nursing: From Then to Now," *Nursing Outlook*, 24 (November 1976): 676–81.

166   Eugene Levine and Evelyn B. Moses, "Registered Nurses Today: A Statistical Profile," *Nursing in the 1980s – Crisis, Opportunities, Challenges*, eds Linda Aiken and Susan Gortner (Philadelphia: J. B. Lippincott, 1982) p. 486. This number comes from the federal

government and may be accurate but there are wide variations in the counts of these specialty groups.

167   Historian and physician Joel Howell's analysis of the medical story uses cardiology as an example. J. Howell, "The Changing Face of Twentieth-Century American Cardiology," *Annals of Internal Medicine*, 105 (November 1986): 772–82.

168   Claire Fagin, "Nursing's Pivotal Role in American Health Care," in Linda Aiken and Susan Gortner (eds), *Nursing in the 1980s*, pp. 459–502. This is one of several essays by this author linking the productivity of nurses and their safe care results with the problems of financing American health care.

169   Mathy Mezey, "The Future of Primary Care and Nurse Practitioners," in *Nurses, Nurse Practitioners, the Evolution of Primary Care* (Boston and Toronto: Little, Brown and Company, 1986) pp. 37–51.

170   Donna Diers, "Nurse-Midwives and Nurse Anesthetists: The Cutting Edge in Specialist Practice," in *Charting Nursing's Future: Agenda for the 1990s*, ed. Linda Aiken and Claire Fagin (Philadelphia: J. B. Lippincott, 1992) pp. 159–80, makes this point very well, noting the substitutability of nurse-midwives for obstetricians and the complementarity of nurse anesthetists to surgeons. The significance of this issue is evidenced by oral testimony before the 1981 National Commission on Nursing when nurse–physician relationships were cited as of major importance by physicians and nursing service administrators. National Commission on Nursing, "Summary of the Public Hearings," [sponsored by] American Hospital Association, Hospital Research and Education Trust, and American Hospital Supply Corporation.

171   In 1980 there were 67,000 nurses holding the master's or doctoral degree; in 1986, 100,100 nurses held master's or doctoral degrees. *Health, United States* (Washington DC: Public Health Service, 1988). In 1992 Health and Human Services reported 150,728 master's and doctorally prepared nurses. "RN Population Grows to 2.2 Million: Nurses Age a Bit but Work More," *American Journal of Nursing* (October 1994): 68. The demand for the year 2000 is predicted to be 392,000 nurses with master's or doctoral training. Health Resources and Services Administration, *Seventh Report to the President and Congress on the Status of Health Personnel in the United States*, US Department of Health and Human Services, March 1990, pp. viii, 39.

172   In 1981 WICHE (Western Interstate Commission for Higher Education) predicted a surplus of 332,000 nurses with associate degrees or hospital diplomas and a deficit of 506,000 nurses with baccalaureate or higher degrees. It determined that the real shortage of nurses [was at] bachelor's, master's and doctoral levels. Problems of clinical competence and high turnover in hospital nursing were reiterated in testimony. Summary of Public Hearings, National Commission on Nursing.

173 By the mid-1980s the number of patient days spent in nursing homes far exceeded [nearly doubled] the number of patient days spent in hospitals. National Center for Health Statistics, *Advance Data from Vital and Health Statistics*, No. 42 (Hyattsville, MD: Public Health Service, 1987).

174 Institute of Medicine, Committee on Nursing and Nursing Education, *Nursing and Nursing Education: Public Policies and Private Actions* (Washington DC: National Academy Press, 1983).

175 Ibid., p. xv.

176 Ibid., p. 8.

177 Ibid., p. 11.

178 Ibid., p. 2.

179 The Secretary's Commission on Nursing, *Final Report* (Washington DC: US Department of Health and Human Services, 1988).

180 See Margaret McClure et al., *Magnet Hospitals – Attraction and Retention of Professional Nurses* (Kansas City: American Academy of Nursing, 1985).

181 Donald Yett, "Yes Virginia, There is a Shortage of Nurses – But it is Not Quite as Simple as All That," Second Conference on the Economics of Health, Baltimore, MD, 1963.

182 Stuart H. Altman, *Present and Future Supply of Registered Nurses* (Washington DC: US Department of Health, Education and Welfare, 1971) pp. 3, 9.

183 Linda H. Aiken, "Breaking the Shortage Cycles," in *Nurses for the Future: A Special Supplement. American Journal of Nursing*, 87 (1987): 1616–20.

184 Eli Ginzberg, "Health Personnel: The Challenges Ahead," *Frontiers of Health Services Management*, 7 (Winter 1990): 3–20.

185 Linda H. Aiken, "Increasing the Supply of Health Personnel: What has been Gained?" *Frontiers of Health Services Management*, 7 (Winter 1990): 23–7.

186 Karen Zander, "The 1990's: Core Values, Core Change," *Frontiers of Health Service Management*, 7 (Winter 1990): 28–32.

187 William A. Knaus et al., "An Evaluation of Outcome from Intensive Care in Major Medical Centers," *Annals of Internal Medicine*, 104 (1986): 410–18.

188 Claire M. Fagin, "The Visible Problems of an 'Invisible' Profession: The Crisis and Challenge for Nursing," *Inquiry*, 24 (Summer 1987): 119–126, p. 125. Fagin reiterates this concern in several subsequent articles as the imbalance continues. The most recent is Claire Fagin and Joan Lynaugh, "Reaping the Rewards of Radical Change: A New Agenda for Nursing Education, *Nursing Outlook*, 40 (September/October 1992): 213–20.

189 American Association of Colleges of Nursing, *News*, 31 December 1994.

190 AACN, *News*, 31 December 1994. Investment is the right word

when speaking of master's education. The majority (70 percent) of master's students in nursing pay their own way and study part-time.

191 Linda Aiken and Marla Salmon, "Health Care Workforce Priorities: What Nursing Should Do Now," *Inquiry*, 31 (Fall 1994): 318–29. L. Aiken and Marnie Gwyther, "Medicare Funding of Nurse and Paramedical Education" (Philadelphia: Center for Health Services and Policy Research, 1994).

192 One mark of the irritation of nurses is the success of the new journal *Revolution – The Journal of Nurse Empowerment*. This journal sets as its target a "revolt against the system that consistently denigrates, devalues, insults, and exploits registered nurses – to the detriment of patient safety and health in the name of self-interested economic profits." *Revolution* (Fall 1994), p. 3.

193 Mary Naylor, Dorothy Brooten, et al., "Comprehensive Discharge Planning for Hospitalized Elderly: A Randomized Clinical Trial," *Annals of Internal Medicine*, 120 (1994): 999–1006. This study illustrates the ways that well prepared nurses can provide services to allow early patient transition from hospital to home which are low-risk and low-cost.

194 "Tough Road Ahead for Nurses' Panel," *Modern Health Care* (18 July 1994), p. 18.

195 Ibid.

196 John Eisenberg, "If Trickle-Down Physician Workforce Policy Failed, Is the Choice Now between the Market and Government Regulation?" *Inquiry*, 28 (Fall 1994): 241–9.

197 Herman Finer. *Administration and the Nursing Services* (New York: Macmillan, 1952), p. 124.

198 Ibid., p. 124.

199 Steven Shortell, Robin R. Gillies, and Kelly J. Devers, "Reinventing the American Hospital," *Milbank Quarterly*, 73 (1995): 131–60, provides a useful overview and analysis of the effect of system development on hospitals.

200 Nursing salaries in home care are competitive with hospital nursing salaries. Most home-care agencies receive a significant portion of their revenues from Medicare and therefore can pass through competitive employee salaries and benefits.

201 Rosemary Stevens, *In Sickness and In Wealth*, p. 355.

202 James R. Knickman et al., "The Potential for Using Non-Physicians to Compensate for the Reduced Availability of Residents," *Academic Medicine*, 67 (July 1992): 429–38.

203 This can be problematic. For instance, in a detailed discussion of the need to revitalize primary care, the author seemed unaware of the twenty-five-year primary-care experience of nurse practitioners and nurse-midwives. Gordon T. Moore, "The Case of the Disappearing Generalist," *Milbank Quarterly*, 70 (1992): 361–79.

204 See, for example, Ellen Rudy and Abe Grenvik, "Future of Critical Care," *American Journal of Critical Care*, 1 (July 1992): 33–7.
205 Janna L. Dieckmann, "From Almshouse to City Nursing Home, Philadelphia's Riverview Home for the Aged, 1945–1965," *Nursing History Review*, 1 (January 1993): 217–28; Joan Lynaugh, *The Community Hospitals of Kansas City, Missouri, 1870–1915* (New York: Garland Press, 1989); for rejection of tuberculous patients see Barbara Bates, *Bargaining for Life – A Social History of Tuberculosis, 1876–1938* (Philadelphia: University of Pennsylvania Press, 1992).
206 Steven A. Schroeder, "Clinical Intensity Versus Cost Containment," and Mitchell Rabkin, "The Hospital as a Social System: New Roles and Relationships," in *Transactions and Studies of the College of Physicians of Philadelphia*, 12 (June 1990): 207–25. Dr Rabkin's discussion of the contemporary hospital scene is cosmopolitan and comprehensive.
207 Stevens, *In Sickness and in Wealth*, p. 364.

Index